Securing Health

This book offers a critical inquiry into the framing of health and disease as a security issue.

In particular, the book examines what happens in the United Nations when the ostensibly 'low' politics of global health meet the 'high' politics of security, and when the logic of security comes to shape global health initiatives. It offers a critical re-assessment of efforts in the United Nations system to position HIV as a security threat with the hope that this would attract greater attention and resources for the global HIV response. The book advances securitization theory by presenting a new framework for studying HIV as a policy process, uniting several theoretical strands into a single, powerful model for empirical application. It uses this model to draw attention to important, understudied aspects of HIV securitization, including the role played by discourses about Africa, and the evolution of ideas about HIV and security as actors learned over time. On the basis of this empirically grounded assessment of how securitization works as a theory and a political strategy, the book suggests that securitization is inherently limited, and perhaps dangerous, as a strategy for 'securing' social change.

This book will be of much interest to students of critical security studies, global health, development studies, and IR in general.

Suzanne Hindmarch is Assistant Professor of political science at the University of New Brunswick, Canada.

Routledge Critical Security Studies series

Titles in this series include:

Securing Health

HIV and the limits of securitization

Suzanne Hindmarch

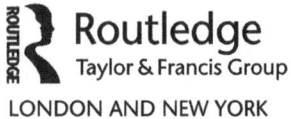

Routledge
Taylor & Francis Group

LONDON AND NEW YORK

First published 2016 by Routledge

2 Park Square, Milton Park, Abingdon, Oxfordshire OX14 4RN

52 Vanderbilt Avenue, New York, NY 10017

Routledge is an imprint of the Taylor & Francis Group, an informa business

First issued in paperback 2020

British Library Cataloguing-in-Publication Data
A catalogue record for this book is available from the British Library

Library of Congress Cataloging-in-Publication Data
Names: Hindmarch, Suzanne, author.
Title: Securing health : HIV and the limits of securitization /
Suzanne Hindmarch.
Other titles: Routledge critical security studies series.
Description: Abingdon, Oxon ; New York, NY : Routledge, 2016. | Series:
Routledge critical security studies series | Includes bibliographical
references and index.
Identifiers: LCCN 2015046763| ISBN 9781138860384 (hbk) |
ISBN 9781315716480 (ebk)
Subjects: | MESH: United Nations. | HIV Infections | Security Measures |
Health Policy | International Agencies
Classification: LCC RA643.86.A35 | NLM WC 503 | DDC 362.19697/92–dc23
LC record available at http://lccn.loc.gov/2015046763

ISBN: 978-1-138-86038-4 (hbk)
ISBN: 978-0-367-59668-2 (pbk)

Typeset in Times New Roman
by Wearset Ltd, Boldon, Tyne and Wear

Contents

Illustrations

Figures

Tables

Acknowledgements

I have been fortunate to benefit from the help of many people while writing this book. First, I would like to thank all those whom I interviewed for generously sharing their time, insights and frank reflections. Although our conclusions about HIV securitization may differ in some cases, I have tremendous respect and appreciation for their work supporting those most affected by HIV, armed conflict and humanitarian emergencies. For their thoughtful comments on earlier versions of this manuscript, I am grateful to Antoinette Handley, Matt Hoffmann, Dickson Eyoh, Nancy Bertoldi and Michael C. Williams. I am also grateful to Stefan Elbe, as well as many discussants at ISA conferences over the years, for feedback and suggestions about how to approach the questions at the core of the book. The comments of two anonymous reviewers were very helpful and improved the manuscript considerably. This book has its roots in my doctoral research and fieldwork, which was financially supported by Ontario Graduate Scholarships. At the other end of this lengthy process, I thank Andrew Humphrys and Hannah Ferguson at Routledge and Hannah Riley at Wearset for seeing this book through to publication. I also thank Sandra Stafford for copyediting and Angela Pietrobon for indexing the manuscript. For their encouragement and support throughout, deepest thanks to my friends, and family including Marilyn and Brian Hindmarch, Kristie Dehid, and Tyler Somers.

Abbreviations

AIDS	Acquired Immune Deficiency Syndrome
ARV	Antiretroviral
ASCI	AIDS, Security and Conflict Initiative
ASO	AIDS Service Organization
CMA	Civil–Military Alliance to Combat HIV and AIDS
CS	Copenhagen School
CSS	Critical Security Studies
DDR	Disarmament, Demobilization and Reintegration
DPKO	Department of Peacekeeping Operations
DRC	Democratic Republic of the Congo
ECOSOC	Economic and Social Council of the United Nations
GPA	Global Programme on AIDS
HIV	Human Immunodeficiency Virus
IDU	Injecting drug user
IO	International organization
IR	International Relations
JUNTA	Joint United Nations Team on AIDS
MSM	Men who have sex with men
NGO	Non-governmental organization
OCHA	Office for the Coordination of Humanitarian Affairs
P5	The five permanent members of the United Nations Security Council (China, France, Great Britain, the Russian Federation, USA)
PEP	Post-exposure prophylaxis
PHA	Person living with HIV/AIDS
SEA	Sexual Exploitation and Abuse
SHR	Security and Humanitarian Response
SSR	Security Sector Reform
STI	Sexually transmitted infection
TAC	Treatment Action Campaign
TB	Tuberculosis
UN	United Nations
UNAIDS	Joint United Nations Programme on HIV/AIDS

UNDP	United Nations Development Programme
UNGASS	United Nations General Assembly Special Session
UNHCR	United Nations High Commissioner for Refugees
UNFPA	United Nations Population Fund
UNSC	United Nations Security Council
VCCT	Voluntary Confidential Counselling and Testing
VCT	Voluntary Counselling and Testing
WFP	World Food Programme
WHO	World Health Organization

1 Introduction

HIV and securitization as a transformative strategy in global health

We live in a world of apparently finite resources and infinite need. Yet decisions about resource allocation are rarely a problem of absolute material constraints; more usually, the greatest challenge is not the total available amount of resources, but how and to whom those resources are distributed. Deliberations about which and whose issues matter most, and therefore have the greatest claim to attention and resources, are intensely political and significantly shape resource distribution. In global health, the distribution of resources including money and medicine, and the inequities produced by unequal access to these resources, are literally a matter of life and death. How, then, to draw attention and resources to a particular global health issue, or to incite particular policy and programmatic action? More fundamentally, how might resource allocation, and the systems that determine how and to whom political attention is given and life-saving resources granted, be transformed to produce a more just world?

This book examines the efficacy and transformative potential of one strategy for attracting attention and resources to global health: securitization, defined as a move in which actors in a position of authority construct an issue as an existential threat, circumventing the deliberative processes of 'normal politics' and triggering emergency action in the form of rule-breaking threat response (Buzan, Wæver, & de Wilde, 1998). It is a critical inquiry into what happens to health and disease when they are constructed in security terms in the current, actually existing international system: when the ostensibly 'low' politics of global health meet the 'high' politics of international security, and when the logic of securitization comes to shape global health initiatives. The book undertakes this inquiry by examining the effort of a small number of elite actors in the United Nations system to position HIV as a security threat and place it on the agenda of the United Nations Security Council (UNSC), with the aim of increasing global HIV funding and treatment access. These actors' decision to securitize HIV was a departure from the strategies previously employed by activists in the global HIV response, whose calls for urgent action (as will be discussed below) did not rely on the language of security or the logic of securitization. It also represented a departure from previous international security practice, marking the first time the UNSC had ever identified a disease as a security threat. Yet in its assumption that security holds unique power to attract attention and catalyse urgent action, and that securitization can therefore be an effective means of attracting resources and producing political change, the decision reflects a widely-held belief.

Assumptions about the power and political potential of security and securitization significantly shape security studies theory,[1] and the practices of actors seeking resources or, more generally, swift and decisive political action. These assumptions are politically and empirically as well as theoretically consequential: HIV securitization, and the interventions such securitization authorizes or conversely fails to achieve, has profound human consequences for the approximately 36 million people living with HIV (AIDSInfoOnline (UNAIDS-supported data repository), 2015) and the much larger number of people affected by it. In addition to suggesting to policy-makers and community activists alike how we ought to understand and respond to the global HIV pandemic, beliefs about the efficacy and ethics of securitization also have much wider relevance for other advocates seeking strategies to advance redistributive or transformative agendas in support of social justice. They are assumptions that therefore warrant closer scrutiny – as do the UNSC sessions themselves, which remain an oft-cited but sometimes misunderstood instance of securitization. Careful examination of the UNSC's securitization of HIV can provide an empirically grounded way in to understanding how securitization works as a theory and a political strategy, and in so doing, enables assessment of some widely held beliefs about power, security, securitization, and political change.

This book, then, has three central aims. The first is to advance securitization theory by proposing a framework to support comprehensive empirical examination of securitization. The book presents a new framework for studying securitization as a policy process, historically produced and organizationally situated, that encompasses discourses, bureaucratic practices, exception and routine, and that is characterized by change as well as continuity over time. Theoretically, the framework unites several strands of securitization theory, levels of analysis and categories of actors in a single framework. Analytically, conceptualising securitization as a series of policy stages enables structured, systematic tracing of the origins, evolution and effects of securitization at multiple levels and points in time, with particular focus on the nature and form of meaning-making contests at each stage. The framework holds potentially wide utility for studying 'real world' securitizations, and is intended to contribute to ongoing conversations about securitization theory and its empirical applications. Readers whose primary interest is in the global response to HIV, or in the utility of securitization as a social justice strategy, will also find the framework a useful model with which to investigate instances of securitization; in this respect, the book is an example of what securitization theory can offer to those with an empirical interest in how security is invoked, with what consequences, in 'real world' cases.

This leads to the book's second aim, which is to trace, using this framework, how the UNSC's HIV securitization unfolded, and what its consequences have been. The overarching argument is that the UNSC sessions were neither the game-changer some participants had hoped they would be, nor were they a failed securitization. Rather, they were at once exceptional and limited, in ways that suggest inherent constraints to the transformative potential of securitization. The book shows that the UNSC sessions and resulting resolutions had significant impact, but in a different form and location than is usually recognized: not in the global HIV response writ large, but in peacekeeping missions, in the UN system itself, and in the epistemic community of HIV and security analysts and practitioners. Additionally, this securitization was not, as is sometimes suggested, simply driven by the US. Rather, there was a distinct international-level move to securitize HIV, and this securitization itself has evolved significantly over time. These arguments are developed by carefully tracing the trajectory of the UNSC's HIV securitization from its origins in historically-produced discourses, to meaning-making contests in the UNSC's initial debates in 2000, to the evolution and significant revision of the idea 'HIV is a security threat' over the next decade. For security and securitization theorists, the analysis provides granular exploration of the dynamics of securitization as a policy process, showing how discourses and bureaucratic practices work in a specific context and over time to produce securitizations, and how actor learning can produce change in securitizations' meaning and content. For readers with an interest in the practical politics of HIV and social justice, the analysis usefully illuminates how and why securitization is limited as a strategy for catalysing social change. For both audiences, this empirical analysis provides a critical re-evaluation of the origins, dynamics and consequences of the UNSC's securitization of HIV.

The third aim of the book is to, from empirical analysis, derive a normative assessment of the ethics and efficacy of securitization as a political strategy. The argument is that securitization holds inherent limitations, largely due to its reliance on threat construction and resulting binary us/Other relations, which create difference, and then hierarchies based on this difference. This produces consistent constraints that shape all subsequent threat response, making securitization an ineffective and dangerous strategy for social change. On this basis, while not claiming to offer definitive answers or solutions, the book proposes that to achieve lasting change in global health resource distribution, we require not securitization strategies, but rather desecuritization efforts that make normal politics itself the site and object of emancipatory praxis. This normative assessment is likely to be of interest to theorists and practitioners with an interest in social justice, emancipation, and strategies and theories of political change.

In sum, this is a book about securitization, and how it works as a theory, policy process and political strategy. It is a book about security-in-use: how security in this instance was understood, operationalized and enacted by people working in and around the UN system in what became, following the UNSC sessions in 2000, the UN's 'security response' to HIV. And it is a book about one facet of the global response to HIV: especially, what happened when much larger claims about HIV as an urgent problem requiring exceptional response were interpreted by, and addressed in and through, the predominantly military-focused international security sector. To situate the arguments that unfold over the rest of the book, the remainder of this chapter briefly outlines the empirical case, locates the UNSC's treatment of HIV in the larger context of the global HIV response, and establishes the book's foundational premises and theoretical orientation.

HIV securitization in the UN system

The UNSC's January 2000 session is often cited as a pivotal moment in which HIV and security concerns were brought together in a novel manner that transformed them both. But this elides that the events of 2000 were not simply a securitization of *HIV*. The UNSC initially considered HIV as a threat to peace, security and development *in Africa*, the continent most severely and disproportionately affected by HIV.[2] Using his prerogative as UNSC president (a position that rotates among UNSC members), US Ambassador Richard Holbrooke declared that January 2000 would be the "month of Africa", and that the first session would be devoted to a consideration of HIV's impact on the continent. In this initiative, he was supported and influenced by UNAIDS executive director Peter Piot, who was seeking to draw attention and funding to the global HIV response. The debate was a historic first for the UNSC, garnering considerable political and popular press attention. The session was characterized by far-reaching discussion about the impact of HIV on Africa, calls for improved treatment access on the continent and elsewhere in the global South, and observations about the mutually reinforcing relationship between poverty, underdevelopment, violence and the spread of HIV. It did not however culminate in any action or policy directives.

The UNSC's first HIV-related resolution was passed in July 2000, and it reflected a crucial reframing of the problem: from an initial focus on HIV's impact on Africa, the July 2000 session was far more narrowly focused on the impact of HIV on *peacekeeping*. The outcome, Resolution 1308, called for HIV prevention programmes for peacekeepers as a means of addressing the putative threat posed by HIV. The provision of condoms to peacekeepers was a very limited response when compared to the policy problem as originally stated: that is, HIV's impact on security and development in Africa. It certainly did nothing to address the significant, complex health and development issues that had been raised in the January UNSC sessions. However, having been given a mandate to address HIV in peacekeeping, UN actors tasked with implementing this 'security response to HIV' developed programming that, as this book shows, has come to constitute exceptional reach into territories and peacekeepers' bodies – even as it has done little to reach those most vulnerable to HIV.

There followed two sessions in 2001 and 2005 to update the UNSC on progress in implementing Resolution 1308, after which HIV was not discussed again until June 2011, when a second resolution addressing HIV was passed. Resolution 1983 linked HIV to conflict, post-conflict and peacebuilding, foregrounded the relationship between HIV, gender and sexual violence, and repositioned peacekeepers from vectors of HIV transmission to HIV educators, but made no mention of the especially severe impact of HIV on African states and communities. It expressed a very different understanding of how, why and to whom HIV was a security threat than had been articulated in the initial securitizing moves of 2000, and endorsed a far more expansive set of UN-led programming activities with uniformed services and humanitarian populations, and in conflict and post-conflict states.

From the outset, then, HIV securitization efforts reflected two quite different concerns: the health of Africa and Africans living with HIV on the one hand, and the integrity and effectiveness of peacekeeping missions on the other. The sessions began with evident confusion about the meaning of 'security' and 'threat', and how each of these concepts related to HIV – that is, whether HIV was a threat to states or to people, and whether it was threatening to African or non-African states or people or both. Additionally, once the focus shifted to peacekeepers, UNSC session participants showed no consensus about whether by 'peacekeepers' they meant troops from African states, troops serving in African missions, or all peacekeepers. Peacekeepers were mainly discussed as threatening vectors of HIV transmission in 2000, but by 2011 they were reconstructed as HIV educators. Iterations of HIV securitization in 2000 and 2011 also expressed quite different understandings of the HIV-security relationship and its connection to, variously, Africa, peacekeeping, gender, and sexual violence, indicating the significant evolution of this securitization over time.

This points to the contentious, contested and perpetually unstable meaning of 'HIV is a security threat', suggesting that HIV securitization has been a dynamic, ongoing meaning-making process. At the same time, securitizing actors' almost immediate empirical slippage from positioning HIV as a security problem to locating that problem in the security *sector*, specifically in peacekeeping, suggests that securitizing moves, although theorized as entailing the radical construction of security (Buzan et al., 1998), are in practice limited by and reflective of security-in-use; that is, the prior norms and understandings that work in a given context to define what security means, which populations and sectors fall within the boundaries of security, and who has the authority to act on security matters.

HIV securitization in the UN system of course took place against the backdrop of much larger political shifts. In particular, a vocal, well-organized transnational HIV/AIDS activist movement, calling for greater political action and financial investments to address HIV, had gained significant momentum over the mid- to late 1990s. By 2000 this movement had contributed to a widespread general sense that HIV was an exceptional global problem (Ingram, 2013), if not specifically a security threat, and this general sense of urgency undoubtedly contributed to the impetus for the UNSC sessions. Activist mobilization in support of universal treatment access would eventually trigger significant transformation in the global response, especially by successfully challenging pharmaceutical patents on, and prohibitively high pricing of, ARVs (Gray, 2012; Kapstein & Busby, 2013; Mugyenyi, 2008; Smith & Siplon, 2006); it was a mobilization that would ultimately have much greater effect on the global response than securitization efforts and the resulting 'security response to HIV' in the UN system.

This does not mean that the more localized securitization of HIV as it manifested in the UN system, international security sector and peacekeeping was unimportant or inconsequential. On the contrary, careful examination of this case suggests that securitizations can simultaneously have limited macro- or systems-level impact, while still producing exception, excess and deeply ethically problematic results that less granular analysis will overlook. In the case of the UNSC's HIV securitization, both of these effects are significant: not only did this securitization fail to trigger substantive action on the policy problem it ostensibly set out to address – the devastating impact of HIV on, and lack of treatment access in, Africa – but it produced exceptional practices within UN-led programming in the security sector that may not, themselves, effectively prevent HIV among peacekeepers or improve access to HIV support and treatment.

Interpreting international HIV securitization

Following Resolution 1308, the HIV-security nexus emerged as an area of interest in political science.[3] To some observers, the UNSC's construction of HIV as a security threat seemed a textbook case of securitization, a theory introduced by the Copenhagen School (CS) only a few years earlier (Buzan et al., 1998) (though as discussed below, it is not always clear that some of the diverse HIV-security linkages glossed as HIV securitization actually meet the criteria laid out by securitization theory). There is emerging consensus about some aspects of the UNSC sessions and HIV securitization, but other aspects are still debated, or have received little attention.

First, while HIV securitization in the UN system reflected a widely-held sentiment that HIV required urgent action, activists were not clamouring for HIV to be discussed by the Security Council, nor were most of the Council's permanent members keen to discuss HIV (Prins, 2004; Rushton, 2010; Sternberg, 2002). Certainly, some actors saw this as a pragmatic move (Elbe, 2009; Prins, 2004), thought to be effective at mobilising resources for the global response; and certainly, US Ambassador Holbrooke, as then-president of the UNSC, had an important role to play in placing HIV on the UNSC agenda in spite of P5 resistance (McInnes & Rushton, 2013). But while this may explain actors' beliefs about what is politically pragmatic or desirable, it does not explain the origins of those beliefs, or how and why those beliefs gain traction. It raises the question of how the idea 'HIV is a security threat' became thinkable in the first place: beyond and before the deliberate actions of Holbrooke and other securitizing actors, which were only the proximate cause of HIV securitization in the UNSC, how did it become possible for HIV to be plausibly securitized, when so many other devastating diseases were not? What perceived properties of HIV, and of Africa, worked to make the idea 'HIV is a security threat' an intelligible and seemingly compelling, if contested, proposition?

This book explores these questions by delving more deeply into the discourses about Africa, HIV and security that, I argue, are what made HIV securitization 'thinkable'. By attending to how Africa was invoked and the work this invocation did, we can uncover the crucial discursive role of Africa in international HIV securitization, and the material impact of this securitization on African states and people, some of whom (including those most vulnerable to and affected by HIV) were not reached by this securitized response, and others of whom (by virtue of their role as peacekeepers) were significantly impacted. We also, by focusing on international actors' efforts to promote, and influence the meaning of, the idea 'HIV is a security threat', can distinguish some uniquely international-level elements of this securitization.

Additionally, analysis to date has focused almost exclusively on Resolution 1308 and the events of 2000 (Elbe, 2002, 2003, 2009; McInnes, 2006; McInnes & Rushton, 2013; Rushton, 2010); Resolution 1983, which articulated a very different understanding of HIV and security (one in which Africa was not mentioned at all) has not received significant scholarly attention. This is understandable, as most of this work was written before the UNSC's return to HIV in 2011. But it has perhaps created the impression, for casual readers, that international HIV securitization occurred in and shortly after 2000, and that the meaning and content of this securitization has since been stable. Consequently, the significant evolution of ideas about HIV, Africa and security from 2000 to 2011 has not been recognized. As this book shows, this evolution has much to tell us about how actor learning can produce change in securitizations over time, and therefore how we might theorize and empirically study the process and effects of securitization.

Finally, with respect to outcomes, there continue to be quite different interpretations of the impact, efficacy and ethics of HIV securitization. McInnes and Rushton contend that Resolution 1308 did not directly produce significant increases in funding for the global HIV response, and that the most significant gains in the global response have not relied on the invocation of security (McInnes & Rushton, 2013; Rushton, 2010). They therefore suggest that Resolution 1308 represents at best a partial securitization (McInnes & Rushton, 2010). Elbe (2006, 2009) reaches a different conclusion – which, to be clear, is primarily in support of a theoretical argument about the governmentalization of security, not an empirical argument about HIV. Elbe suggests that while there are potential dangers to securitizing HIV, and that to mitigate these dangers it would be preferable for actors to treat HIV not as a threat, but a complex problem with a security dimension, HIV securitization has, in practice, attracted attention and triggered political action without having significant negative impact such as increased stigma, discrimination or curtailment of human rights. Seckinelgin (2012), in contrast, suggests that these studies fail to consider the complexities of lived experience. He finds securitization an inadequate policy and analytical frame through which to address the lived realities of HIV vulnerability, especially those of women, in conflict and post-conflict states. Importantly, Elbe and Seckinelgin use 'securitization' to refer, in a general and capacious way, to HIV-security linkages, and neither makes extensive use of securitization theory in their analysis. This raises the questions: what are the parameters of HIV securitization, and how should securitization theory be applied to empirical instances of efforts to construct HIV as a security issue? I will return to these questions shortly.

When our analytical gaze is directed at the global HIV response writ large, all of these authors are correct. Resolution 1308 did, as McInnes and Rushton observe, have limited material impact on the global response. In general, Elbe is correct that international efforts to link HIV and security seem not to have triggered additional widespread exceptional practices, discrimination, and curtailment of rights (though his argument that securitization cannot be said to have caused these practices because HIV-related stigma, discrimination, quarantine and travel restrictions were in place in many states before international-level HIV securitizing moves (Elbe, 2009, pp. 92–95), may actually suggest the power of national and sub-national securitizations, which are mainly left out of his global-level analysis). And Seckinelgin is correct that few studies of securitization have been grounded in local-level consideration of lived experiences, and this is a serious deficit in much IR theorising.

But this book argues that, first, if we examine the discourses about Africa from and through which international HIV securitization emerged, we find that "biopolitical racism", i.e. the casting of Africa and Africans as diseased and dangerous (Elbe, 2005), and HIV-related stigma constructing people with HIV as threats (McInnes & Rushton, 2010), are not simply potential risks that *might* result from securitization; on the contrary, these were foundational to HIV securitization. Additionally, when we focus our attention on the security sector and peacekeeping – the sector most directly and deeply implicated in the UNSC's HIV securitization – and if we ground our study in careful, situated analysis of the UN bureaucracies within which HIV and security programming originates, of the programming itself, and of the peace missions and peacekeepers that are the ultimate objects of this programming, we find significant localized impact. This impact includes precisely the circumvention of debate and the illiberal, exceptional practices predicted by securitization theory. HIV securitization has had tremendous impact within UN-led work in the international security sector, where the 'security response' to HIV has been characterized by exceptional incursions into territories and bodies, and expansion of these exceptional practices over time. Yet it has also failed to meaningfully address or improve the lives of those most affected by and vulnerable to HIV, including the women represented in Seckinelgin's study and the African populations who were invoked to justify HIV securitization. In sum, when we shift our analytical gaze, we find that the UNSC's HIV securitization has produced at once exceptional and limited effects, both of which have been problematic.

We also find that, when securitization is reimagined as a policy process, securitization theory is capable of precisely the grounded analysis called for by Seckinelgin, who asks us to begin not at the abstract level of the international, but with concrete, specific political events and the lived experiences of people.[4] Yet international-level securitizations do not emerge as an abstract, ungrounded view from nowhere – they do not spring fully formed from the minds of policymakers like Athena from Zeus' forehead. Securitizations, even at elite levels of global politics, emerge intersubjectively, from the perspectives, lived experiences, and interactions among actors who are also "real people in real places" (Booth, 2005, p. 275). To understand HIV securitization we also need, therefore, situated empirical analysis of another sort: precisely at the level of international policy, in elite and bureaucratic spheres of policy development and implementation. This book is not an ethnography, but its granular study of HIV securitization in the bureaucratic context of the UN system can complement ethnographic studies of local, lived experience by showing how international actors and organizations interpret HIV, security and 'the local', and how these interpretations then shape the policies and programmes with such power to influence, from a distance, the daily lives of people affected by HIV.

All of this points to a further set of unanswered questions about the outcomes of HIV securitization: how should we understand the at once limited and exceptional practices produced by HIV securitization, and the evolution and durability of the idea 'HIV is a security threat' over time? How should we reconcile the transformative aims of some of the architects of this HIV securitization with its narrow outcomes, particularly given the ostensible power of security to attract resources, and the pressure to act that had been generated in the larger global response? What do the outcomes of this case suggest about the efficacy of securitization as a strategy for resource acquisition and reallocation? By refocusing analysis directly on the UNSC sessions and their aftermath, and using a new analytical framework treating securitization as a policy process, this book offers a critical rethinking of international HIV securitization and its utility as a social justice tactic.

I want to be clear that while critical of *securitization* as a transformative strategy, this book is neither a critique of HIV-related programming with peacekeepers and uniformed services, nor of those who have pursued securitization as a strategy to transform the global HIV response. UN-led HIV programmes in the security response to HIV may remain ethically problematic (in part because of the securitization logic that has shaped this programming), but they are also necessary; the aim should be to address their ethical shortcomings, not to eliminate the programmes. As for the architects of the UNSC sessions, and the practitioners who continue to hope that invoking security might prove an effective strategy to achieve universal treatment access, these were and are deeply committed individuals who have sought, often in the face of maddening state and public indifference, a better and more just response to a disease that continues disproportionately to affect, and to kill, the most marginalized and vulnerable among us. Invoking the rhetoric of security and the logic of securitization seemed for many, in 2000, an empirically accurate description of the impact of HIV on high-prevalence communities, and a morally justified strategy to provoke international action. Pursuing securitization as a strategy to transform the global response was also the only way to discover the efficacy of that strategy. Now, almost two decades after the first UNSC sessions and five years after the second sessions, it is time to take stock of what they, and international HIV securitization more broadly, have accomplished. But it is also time for us to examine the impact of this securitization more closely and critically; not to lay blame, but to learn from the past so that we might apply these lessons to future efforts to mobilize for social justice and social change.

Foundational premises: securitization, exceptionalism and the global response to HIV

Empirically-driven debates about how to understand HIV securitization stem from, and are deeply entangled with, questions that cut to the core of securitization theory: how should securitization be defined, and what is its relation to exceptionalism? How should we assess the success, dangers and potential of securitization strategies? And how should the theory be applied to empirical studies of international affairs?

The preceding discussion already indicates that this book rests on some foundational understandings of security, securitization, and exceptionalism, as well as how these manifested in the global HIV response. Most of these theoretical commitments are elaborated in the second and third chapters. Here, however, I briefly outline a few key premises: first, that securitization theory establishes limits, even if these are contested, to what can empirically be defined as a securitization; and second, therefore, not every invocation of urgency, emergency and exceptionalism is a securitization. Third, consequently, this book's interpretation of what is included in international HIV securitization is circumscribed, and does not encompass the entire global HIV activist mobilization. Fourth, while securitization theory is primarily interested in the grammar of security speech, not the presence or absence of the word 'security', when the word is explicitly deployed in securitizing moves, studying its use can provide important insights into how securitizing actors themselves define security.

Securitization: what do you mean?[5]

'Securitization' has entered the political science vernacular, to the extent that it is increasingly used to refer, in a general sense, to 'things discussed in security terms' or 'things identified as requiring exceptional response', by authors who are not actually using securitization theory in their analysis. Consequently, securitization and exceptionalism are sometimes conflated; but the terms are not synonymous. Carefully distinguishing the two concepts shows that securitization entails a distinct logic and produces a specific *type* of exceptionalism, identifiable through particular empirical and rhetorical markers. Where these are absent, there may indeed be exceptionalism, but this should not be conflated with securitization.

The difficulty in determining what 'counts' as a real-world instance of securitization is that different variants of securitization theory have different thresholds for and empirical markers of securitization; there are legitimate differences of opinion about which phenomena, even within the HIV-security nexus, ought to be labelled as 'securitization'. The Copenhagen School (CS) is clear that a threshold of extremity must be reached, while some sociological interlocutors suggest that securitizations can be instantiated through more subtle acts and practices below the level of exception. The theoretical and methodological tensions between these two positions have been thoughtfully explored by Williams (2011) and Balzacq (2011), among others. It is precisely in response to these tensions that this book presents an analytical approach integrating CS and sociological variants of securitization theory into a single policy process framework.

To briefly outline the essence of this approach: I share the view of CS interlocutors who insist on the importance of context (particularly bureaucratic and organizational context) and of approaching securitization as a process unfolding over time. I also share Williams' (2011) concern that without some threshold of extremity and emergency, it is no longer clear how securitization is to be distinguished from any other policy change. Therefore, this book retains the essential empirical and rhetorical definition of securitization proposed by the CS: there must be (1) a speech act that initiates the securitization process, (2) made by an actor in a structural position of authority, who (3) invokes existential threat requiring urgent threat response, which (4) results in exceptional, rule-breaking practices, and usually the circumvention of widespread, open public debate and deliberation (Buzan et al., 1998). I then integrate this into a policy process framework capable of contextualizing and historicizing securitization.

At the core of this approach is the recognition that securitization hinges on the invocation of *threat*, and this is what gives securitization its unique logic, distinguishing it from other invocations of emergency and calls for urgent action. While the tendency of securitization to produce us-them thinking, defensive (Wæver, 1995) or "threat-defense" (Elbe, 2006) responses, and antagonistic relations (Huysmans, 2006) is widely noted, less attention has been given to the dynamics of threat construction, which is sometimes downplayed in favour of a focus on the politics of insecurity, unease, or fear (Huysmans, 2006; Williams, 2011). This book, in contrast, foregrounds the discursive work done by threat itself, arguing that threat construction and response work to produce uniquely hierarchical and oppositional subject identities. Again, this analysis is developed in greater detail in Chapters 2 and 3. For the moment, the key point is that the invocation of threat, and resulting reduction of the world into an 'us' that must be protected from an inherently threatening and less-valued 'Other', gives securitization a specific logic that is not present in every call for urgent action. Threat construction as a rhetorical move then matters politically, because threats can only ever be contained or eradicated; responding to a threat requires a specific, and limited, repertoire of defensive manoeuvres, which restricts the range of policy and programmatic actions that are subsequently possible.

Furthermore, the construction of an existential threat requiring urgent threat response is undertaken with the intent to catalyse rapid action, but the logic of securitization works to produce and enable a specific type of rapid action. What is sought in securitization is not just immediate, decisive response, but also the circumvention of widespread public debate and inclusive deliberative processes, which are necessarily more time consuming. It is a logic that therefore works precisely to circumscribe and restrict decision-making authority; to concentrate greater power and authority in the hands of a select few security actors; and to justify, by pointing to the exigencies of existential threat response, the exceptional, often intrusive and illiberal practices undertaken by these actors.

To be sure, this approach has been critiqued as too narrow, too Schmittian (Roe, 2012), and setting too high a bar for what 'counts' as securitization (Bigo, 2002; Huysmans, 2011). Yet there is utility in maintaining a high, and specific, bar for the exceptionalism that characterizes securitization, and particularly for retaining the requirements that the logic of threat construction and response be present, and that the strategy be undertaken specifically to circumvent debate. The utility is largely empirical and methodological, as Williams (2011, p. 217) has also suggested in his observation that exceptionalism "provide[s] an anchoring device through which 'security' dynamics can be discerned and distinguished from 'normal' change within the policy process". I would further argue that without retaining specific empirical and normative markers for what securitization does (it circumvents debate, concentrates power, and enables intrusive, illiberal practices) and how it works (through the logic of threat construction and response) – that is, without specifying the *type* of exceptionalism it produces – we are left unable to distinguish between securitization and social movement activism.

Every social justice mobilization, from historical campaigns to end slavery and achieve universal suffrage, to contemporary efforts to ban land mines or promote animal rights, to movements including Occupy and Black Lives Matter in the US, Idle No More in Canada, and Rhodes Must Fall and Fees Must Fall in South Africa, is premised on claims that a social group or population is being harmed by something, and that urgent, exceptional action to address this harm is needed. Yet to represent all of these as securitizing moves on the basis that they call for exceptional action poses, first, empirical and analytical problems. If every call for urgent social or political change becomes a securitizing move, then we are left with the same problem that Deudney (1990, p. 464) first identified in efforts to 'widen' security: "[i]f everything that causes a decline in human well-being is labelled a 'security' threat, the term loses any analytical usefulness and becomes a loose synonym of 'bad'." Similarly, if all social movement activism calling for urgent action is defined as securitization, the term is reduced to a loose synonym for 'change'. This renders 'securitization' too capacious a concept to be of analytical use, and returns us, as Williams (2011) argues, to exactly the widening/deepening debates that securitization theory was intended to address.

More importantly, to characterize these forms of mobilization as securitization seems to fundamentally misrepresent the character of most social justice activism, and to misunderstand the logics at the centre of securitization, compared to social justice, strategies. The logic animating social movements is a logic from and on behalf of the social margins of a given political order, undertaken by those not in structural positions of power. At the core of social justice movements are efforts to redefine and expand the boundaries of political community, to break down us/Other and inside/outside binaries, and to render processes of political deliberation and decision-making more inclusive, sometimes quite radically so. This is precisely the opposite of securitization's logic of threat construction followed by rapid, executive action to defend a threatened 'us' from a menacing Other – a logic of exclusion that solidifies (and often shrinks) the boundaries of political community. In sum, social justice movements are transformative efforts, and they demonstrate that rules can be broken and power exercised by collectivities not in structural positions of authority, in ways that do not rely on securitization's binary logic of threat construction and response.

Exceptionalism without securitization: the global response to HIV

Once we have done the conceptual work of disentangling exceptionalism and securitization, we can then see that the global HIV activist movement writ large is best understood as one that, while entailing calls for exceptional action, was not based on the logic of securitization. As I argue elsewhere in this book (see especially Chapter 3), global HIV activist mobilization called for and successfully triggered an exceptional response – reduction in ARV pricing and lifting of patent restrictions – that was not primarily predicated on threat construction or explicit invocation of security concerns, and was not intended to produce illiberal and exclusionary responses. That is, it relied for the most part on neither the logic of securitization nor the language of security.

Most HIV activism in the 1990s invoked the logic and language of human rights (Forman, 2013; Kapstein & Busby, 2013), structural violence and social justice (Gray, 2012; Smith & Siplon, 2006). It included frequent and explicit assertions that a comprehensive response to HIV would require structural transformation to address, *inter alia*, homophobia, gender-based violence, and poverty. In its insistence on the inclusion of people living with HIV in all decisions related to HIV policy and programming, and its use of legal action to promote the rights of the marginalized populations most vulnerable to and affected by HIV (Forman, 2013), the global HIV activist movement sought not to foreclose deliberative processes but to expand and deepen them, and to create more just and inclusive political communities. Whether HIV activism ultimately succeeded in this larger transformative goal can be debated (Farmer, 2008; Ingram, 2013); my intent is not to write a hagiography of the global activist movement, but simply to argue that the logic animating HIV activism has never primarily been the logic of securitization, and that therefore, HIV securitization should be understood as a much more specific and localized phenomenon. International HIV *securitization*, which was premised on threat construction and response, including explicit statements that 'HIV is a security threat', and which was undertaken in part to circumvent debate (especially UN and global health actors' bureaucratic politicking), should not be conflated with the rather different exceptionalism that characterized the global HIV *response* writ large.

Security-in-use: speak security and enter

This brings us, finally, to the extent to which this book considers international HIV securitization through studying use of the word 'security', and especially use of the word to refer specifically to the security sector. Securitization theory is of course mainly interested in the grammar and logic of threat construction, not the actual use of the word 'security'. The CS is clear that actors do not need to literally speak security; they can use other code words recognized, in a given context and by a certain target audience, as synonymous with security (such as talking about dikes in Holland (Buzan et al., 1998, p. 27)).

Still, especially in international-level securitizations where there is often a thinner set of shared meanings and assumptions, actors cannot be assured that, absent explicit use of the term security, their audiences will recognize security speech as such (how many people outside of Holland would recognize discussion of dikes as security speech?). This is especially the case for actors seeking access to bodies, like the UNSC, that are already officially designated as having authority over security matters; security must be spoken in explicit, often very precise ways to gain access to these spaces. Thus, it is often the case that the word 'security' is explicitly deployed in international-level securitizing moves, and the grammar and logic of securitization is articulated through use of the word 'security'. Furthermore, once a matter has been successfully designated as a security threat, subsequent policies, programmes and other responses are also typically designated as 'security' actions.

Where security is explicitly invoked in securitizing moves, careful study of this security-in-use can provide important insights into how the word is defined and understood by securitizing actors, which activities are labelled as 'security' practices, and how this shapes resulting policies, programmes and actions. Such an inquiry is especially important when studying HIV securitization, because at least some of the actors involved in securitizing HIV pursued this strategy in solidarity with the larger HIV activist movement: their intention was to, by casting HIV as an existential threat, circumvent political debates and catalyse rapid reallocation of resources to the global response. They sought, in other words, to bend securitization strategies to emancipatory ends, and they did so by very explicitly invoking the word 'security' to signify existential threat and thereby gain entry to the UNSC, the body within the UN system recognized as having the authority to respond to security threats.

Therefore, much of this book investigates how security was spoken, understood, defined and redefined by actors seeking to securitize HIV. These actors themselves almost immediately conflated security with the security sector; consequently, tracing the empirics of security-in-use has resulted in analysis focusing, in large part, on the security sector. This does not reflect a theoretical commitment or set of assumptions on my part about what security 'really means'; it reflects the empirical reality of security-in-use in the UN system. But that empirical reality does, I argue, suggest significant constraints and limits to securitization (and perhaps to the invocation of security) as a strategy for catalysing emancipatory change.

In this respect, the book can also be read as an intervention into larger debates in security studies about what security can and cannot mean or do. On the one hand we are presented with the claim that security is an inherently negative concept and securitization a dangerous practice, and that projects of emancipation or resistance are best pursued outside of security altogether (Aradau, 2004; Neocleous, 2008; Peoples, 2011). On the other hand are a theoretically diverse set of propositions, advanced both by theorists drawing on securitization theory (Floyd, 2007, 2011; Roe, 2012) and those with a very different conception of security as emancipation (Booth, 2005; Nunes, 2012, 2014), suggesting that security can be a positive concept and site for social justice praxis. These debates have been conducted largely on theoretical terrain, but ultimately need to be adjudicated at the level of practice. It is only from grounded, contextualized analysis of how, by whom, and with what consequences security is invoked and practiced in global politics that we can derive an accurate assessment of the work that security does, for and to whom, and of how malleable 'security' discourses, practices and structures actually are (Browning & McDonald, 2011). Put differently, it is only by comparing our theoretical assumptions against actually-existing security discourse and practice that we can derive normative judgements to then inform future theory-building and political praxis. The policy process model developed in this book provides a framework that can support precisely this type of structured, empirically grounded and contextualized analysis.

Overview of the book

Conceptually, this study might be thought of as an exploded view of securitization as a policy process. Just as exploded view diagrams illustrate how the component pieces of an object fit together, so this book examines the component parts of HIV securitization (discourses, policy, practice, learning, and ideas about HIV, Africa and security), and seeks to explain how they fit together to create a whole that is greater, and different, than the sum of its parts. The book traces the unfolding of HIV securitization as a policy process, beginning with its discursive origins, then examining the securitizing speech acts of 2000 and associated manoeuvring and framing contests, followed by examination of policy implementation, programme development and delivery, the impact of that programming, and the effect that this entire process had on actors' learning over time, especially the role that this learning played in later efforts to rearticulate and revise the meaning of 'HIV is a security threat' in 2011.

Chapter 2 provides an overview of securitization theories, and introduces a new analytical framework, securitization as a policy process, in which several variants of securitization theory are integrated into a single model to support empirical study of the origins, evolution and outcomes of securitization, and normative evaluation of these outcomes. Subsequent chapters each explore a different stage of the policy process to uncover the causes and consequences of HIV securitization.

Chapter 3 explores the discursive, theoretical and normative factors that made HIV as a security threat 'thinkable', focusing on the centrality of 'threat' to discourses of security, HIV and Africa, and contending that these did the ontological work of threat construction prior to the securitizing speech acts made in and by the UNSC. This chapter, by demonstrating the long historical and discursive processes that made HIV securitization possible, is the basis for subsequent arguments about how security speech and practice are constrained by prior discourse – in this case, historically-produced racialized, gendered discourses in which both Africa and HIV were already constructed as threatening.

Chapter 4 turns to the UNSC debates and Resolution 1308 as securitizing speech acts that triggered policy-framing contests in the UN system. The focus here is on the securitizing speech act itself, the point at which the relationship between HIV and security was publicly articulated in the UN in a way that had normative and policy consequences. The chapter identifies two overarching policy narratives, each with different underlying assumptions about how and why HIV is a security threat, arguing that the very factors that made HIV securitization possible in this context also constrained its outcomes.

The remainder of the book moves from securitizing speech acts to security practices, and from policy framing to policy implementation. It unpacks the impact of HIV securitization on the global response to HIV (where effects were minimal) and in the security sector (where exceptional practices are most evident). Chapter 5 considers the policy implementation stage, examining the impact of Resolution 1308 on the organization of HIV and security work in the UN system. It begins with an examination of how actors and agencies interpreted UNSC directives, showing that 'boundary work' in the UN bureaucracy first carved out HIV and security programming as a distinct policy and programmatic niche within the security sector. The chapter then examines how resulting programming, initially narrow in scope, was broadened and deepened over time, enabling greater incursions into previously sovereign and domestic matters at the level of states, and into previously private and autonomous bodily practices and behaviours at the level of uniformed services and the civilians with whom they interact.

Chapter 6 follows the trajectory of HIV and security policy and analysis from Resolution 1308 to Resolution 1983, demonstrating that a combination of actor learning and changes in the policy environment led actors to re-conceive and re-articulate the idea 'HIV is a security threat' in ways that differed significantly from the original securitization – but that still supported the institutionalization of 'everyday exceptionalism', in which the exceptional practices of securitization are bureaucratized and made to seem part of normal, routine programme delivery. Theoretically, the chapter engages the question of how learning can be incorporated into securitization theory to explain the changing content or meaning of a given securitization over time, and the dynamic relationships between security practitioners and analysts.

To conclude the book, Chapter 7 develops a normative critique, based on the preceding empirical analysis, of the limits of securitization as a political strategy.

It inquires whether (and if so, how) desecuritization, with a view to returning the political struggles associated with the HIV response to normal politics, can overcome these limits; it argues that while securitization is limited as a social justice strategy, as a theory it still holds utility for normative and critical projects. Chapter 8 reflects on the book's contributions and the broader implications – for securitization theory and political practice – flowing from the preceding analysis.

Notes

1 Claims that security is the highest of political priorities are widespread across otherwise divergent theoretical perspectives, and are usually presented as facts preceding analysis, not a conclusion following from analysis. These claims include the Copenhagen School's oft-cited statement that " 'security' is the move that takes politics beyond the established rules of the game" (Buzan et al., 1998, p. 22). Beyond securitization theory, others have claimed: "[i]f an issue can be 'securitized' it is the equivalent of playing a trump at cards, for it at once leapfrogs other issues in priority" (Prins, 2004);

> [t]he high political value added of "greater security" has come to trump so easily other available political discourses. Every seasoned political tactician and marketer surely knows that nothing in today's world seems to advance the urgency and importance of a claim more easily than one grafted to security however tenuous such an operation might appear.
>
> (de Larrinaga & Doucet, 2010, p. 1)

"This [using security as a site for emancipatory change] is especially important if security is still that most powerful of political categories – defining political priority, a community's identity and its core values" (McDonald, 2008, p. 580).
2 In 2001 there were approximately 29.4 million people living with HIV (PHAs), of whom approximately 20.9 million were in sub-Saharan Africa. Currently, 40% of the world's HIV+ women live southern Africa, and Africa is also the only continent where the number of new infections among women is higher than among men. There is variation in prevalence rates among southern African states, but the global HIV pandemic is concentrated in and has had the most severe impact upon sub-Saharan Africa, and has particularly affected women and girls (all data from Joint United Nations Programme on HIV/AIDS (UNAIDS), 2012).
3 Initial research was mainly speculative and tentatively accepted that HIV was a security threat (de Waal, 2003; de Waal & Whiteside, 2003; Ostergard Jr. & Tubin, 2004). More recent work debates whether HIV is 'really' a security threat, whether HIV securitization has been successful, and whether the practical limitations and ethical dangers of securitizing HIV are outweighed by the potential benefits securitizing moves can bring (Barnett, 2006; Barnett & Prins, 2006; de Waal, 2006; Elbe, 2005, 2006, 2009; McInnes & Rushton, 2010, 2013; Seckinelgin, 2012; Whiteside, de Waal, & Gebre-Tensae, 2006).
4 This is a project that has long been undertaken by social geographers and anthropologists (Farmer, 2001; Fassin, 2007; Hunter, 2010; Nguyen, 2010), whose work has received regrettably little attention in political science studies of HIV – with Seckinelgin's study being a notable exception.
5 The section title is of course a reference to Huysmans' (1998) article, "Security! What do you mean? From concept to thick signifier."

References

AIDSInfoOnline (UNAIDS-supported data repository). (2015). Estimated global HIV prevalence. Retrieved 5 October 2015 from www.aidsinfoonline.org/devinfo/libraries/aspx/Home.aspx.

Aradau, Claudia. (2004). Security and the democratic scene: desecuritization and emancipation. *Journal of International Relations and Development, 7*(4), 388–413.

Balzacq, Thierry. (2011). A theory of securitization: origins, core assumptions, variants. In Thierry Balzacq (Ed.), *Securitization Theory: How Security Problems Emerge and Dissolve* (pp. 1–30). New York: Routledge.

Barnett, Tony. (2006). A long-wave event. HIV/AIDS, politics, governance and 'security': sundering the intergenerational bond? *International Affairs, 82*(2), 297–313.

Barnett, Tony & Prins, Gwyn. (2006). HIV/AIDS and security: fact, fiction and evidence – a report to UNAIDS. *International Affairs, 82*(2), 359–368.

Bigo, Didier. (2002). Security and immigration: toward a critique of the governmentality of unease. *Alternatives: Global, Local, Political, 27*(1), 63–92.

Booth, Ken. (2005). Beyond critical security studies. In Ken Booth (Ed.), *Critical Security Studies in World Politics* (pp. 259–278). Boulder, CO: Lynne Rienner.

Browning, Christopher S. & McDonald, Matt. (2011). The future of critical security studies: ethics and the politics of security. *European Journal of International Relations, 19*(2), 235–255.

Buzan, Barry, Wæver, Ole, & de Wilde, Jaap. (1998). *Security: A New Framework for Analysis*. Boulder, CO: Lynne Rienner.

de Larrinaga, Miguel & Doucet, Marc G. (2010). Introduction: the global governmentalization of security and the securitization of governance. In Miguel de Larrinaga & Marc G. Doucet (Eds.), *Security and Global Governmentality: Globalization, Governance and the State* (pp. 1–20). New York: Routledge.

de Waal, Alexander. (2003). How will HIV/AIDS transform African governance? *African Affairs, 102*(406), 1–23.

de Waal, Alexander. (2006). *AIDS and Power: Why There Is No Political Crisis – Yet*. New York: Zed Books.

de Waal, Alexander & Whiteside, Alan. (2003). "New variant famine": AIDS and Food crisis in Southern Africa. *The Lancet, 362*(9391), 1234–1237.

Deudney, Daniel. (1990). The case against linking environmental degradation and national security. *Millennium, 19*(3), 461–476.

Elbe, Stefan. (2002). HIV/AIDS and the changing landscape of war in Africa. *International Security, 27*(2), 159–177.

Elbe, Stefan. (2003). *Strategic Implications of AIDS* (Adelphi Paper 357). Oxford: Oxford University Press.

Elbe, Stefan. (2005). AIDS, security, biopolitics. *International Relations, 19*(4), 403–419.

Elbe, Stefan. (2006). Should HIV/AIDS be securitized? The ethical dilemma of linking HIV/AIDS and security. *International Studies Quarterly, 50*(1), 199–144.

Elbe, Stefan. (2009). *Virus Alert: Security, Governmentality, and the AIDS Pandemic*. New York: Columbia University Press.

Farmer, Paul. (2001). *Infections and Inequalities: The Modern Plagues*. Berkeley, CA: University of California Press.

Farmer, Paul. (2008). Challenging orthodoxies: The road ahead for health and human rights. *Health and Human Rights, 10*(1), 5–19.

Fassin, Didier. (2007). *When Bodies Remember: Experiences and Politics of AIDS in*

South Africa (Amy Jacobs & Gabrielle Varro, Trans.). Berkeley, CA: University of California Press.

Floyd, Rita. (2007). Towards a consequentialist evaluation of security: bringing together the Copenhagen and the Welsh Schools of security studies. *Review of International Studies*, (33), 327–350.

Floyd, Rita. (2011). Can securitization theory be used in normative analysis? Towards a just securitization theory. *Security Dialogue*, *42*(4–5), 427–439.

Forman, Lisa. (2013). What contribution have human rights approaches made to reducing AIDS-related vulnerability in sub-Saharan Africa? Exploring the case study of access to antiretrovirals. *Global Health Promotion*, *20*(Supp. 1), 57–63.

Gray, Dylan Mohan (Writer). (2012). *Fire in the Blood*. In Dylan Mohan Gray (producer). Ireland: Dartmouth Films & Films Transit.

Hunter, Mark. (2010). *Love in the Time of AIDS: Inequality, Gender and Rights in South Africa*. Bloomington, IN: Indiana University Press.

Huysmans, Jef. (1998). Security! What do you mean? From concept to thick signifier. *European Journal of International Relations*, *4*(2), 226–255.

Huysmans, Jef. (2006). *The Politics of Insecurity: Fear, Migration and Asylum in the EU*. New York: Routledge.

Huysmans, Jef. (2011). What's in an act? On security speech acts and little security nothings. *Security Dialogue*, *45*(4–5), 371–383.

Ingram, Alan. (2013). After the exception: HIV/AIDS beyond salvation and scarcity. *Antipode*, *45*(2), 436–454.

Joint United Nations Programme on HIV/AIDS (UNAIDS). (2012). Global report: UNAIDS report on the global AIDS epidemic 2012. Geneva: Joint United Nations Programme on HIV/AIDS (UNAIDS).

Kapstein, Ethan B. & Busby, Joshua W. (2013). *AIDS Drugs for All: Social Movements and Market Transformations*. Cambridge, UK: Cambridge University Press.

McDonald, M. (2008). Securitization and the construction of security. *European Journal of International Relations*, *14*(4), 563–587.

McInnes, Colin. (2006). HIV/AIDS and security. *International Affairs*, *82*(2), 315–326.

McInnes, Colin & Rushton, Simon. (2010). HIV, AIDS and security: where are we now? *International Affairs*, *86*(1), 225–245.

McInnes, Colin & Rushton, Simon. (2013). HIV/AIDS and securitization theory. *European Journal of International Relations*, *19*(1), 115–138.

Mugyenyi, Peter. (2008). *Genocide By Denial: How Profiteering from HIV/AIDS Killed Millions*. Kampala: Fountain Publishers.

Neocleous, Mark. (2008). *Critique of Security*. Montreal: McGill-Queen's University Press.

Nguyen, Vinh-Kim. (2010). *The Republic of Therapy: Triage and Sovereignty in West Africa's Time of AIDS*. Durham, NC: Duke University Press.

Nunes, João. (2012). Reclaiming the political: emancipation and critique in security studies. *Security Dialogue*, *43*(4), 345–361.

Nunes, João. (2014). *Security, Emancipation and the Politics of Health: A New Theoretical Perspective*. New York: Routledge.

Ostergard Jr., Robert L. & Tubin, Matthew. (2004). Between state security and state collapse: HIV/AIDS and South Africa's national security. In Nana Poku & Alan Whiteside (Eds.), *The Political Economy of AIDS in Africa*. Aldershot: Ashgate.

Peoples, Columba. (2011). Security after emancipation? Critical theory, violence and resistance. *Review of International Studies*, *37*(3), 1113–1135.

Prins, Gwyn. (2004). AIDS and global security. *International Affairs*, *80*(5), 931–952.

Roe, Paul. (2012). Is securitization a 'negative' concept? Revisiting the normative debate over normal versus extraordinary politics. *Security Dialogue*, *43*(3), 249–266.

Rushton, Simon. (2010). AIDS and international security in the United Nations system. *Health Policy and Planning*, *25*, 495–504.

Seckinelgin, Hakan. (2012). *International Security, Conflict and Gender: 'HIV/AIDS is Another War'*. New York: Routledge.

Smith, Raymond A. & Siplon, Patricia D. (2006). *Drugs Into Bodies: Global AIDS Treatment Activism*. Westport, CT: Praeger.

Sternberg, Steve. (2002, 11 June). The Fixer takes on global AIDS; Richard Holbrooke faces the biggest challenge of his storied career. *USA Today*, D07.

Wæver, Ole. (1995). Securitization and desecuritization. In Ronnie D. Lipschutz (Ed.), *On Security* (pp. 46–86). New York: Columbia University Press.

Whiteside, Alan, de Waal, Alexander, & Gebre-Tensae, Tsadkan. (2006). AIDS, security and the military: a sobering appraisal. *African Affairs*, *105*(419), 201–218.

Williams, Michael C. (2011). The continuing evolution of securitization theory. In Thierry Balzacq (Ed.), *Securitization Theory: How Security Problems Emerge and Dissolve* (pp. 212–222). New York: Routledge.

2 Securitization as a policy process

Securitization theory is characterized by a central tension: it is on the one hand a theory of change, concerned with explaining how security threats are intersubjectively constructed to move issues from normal to securitized politics; yet it has often entailed analytic focus on either the exceptional, temporally-bounded moment of a speech act, or the gradual accretion and repetition of practices. This can have the effect of privileging sedimentation and stability over contestation and change, and can make it difficult to identify the origins of a given securitization and recognize change in the content and meaning of that securitization over time. Exacerbating this difficulty, the theory lacks a well-developed model for empirical application, including one that would support structured, systematic examination of securitization as a historical process. Securitization theory has also given rise to normative disagreements. The original Copenhagen School (CS) architects of the theory, as well as their sociological interlocutors, broadly maintain a normative preference for desecuritization. But others, arguing for the normative rightness of securitization, propose a political project of transforming various social justice goals into security objectives, transforming social ills into security threats, and seeking emancipation via securitization. Securitization theory still requires a stronger analytical framework with which to theorize and empirically examine history and change – that is, to trace the origins, evolution and impact of securitizations over time – and to assess different normative claims about what securitization can do politically.

This chapter therefore proposes the integration of several strands of securitization theory into a single framework to support the systematic, empirically-driven study of securitization as a historical process involving both discursive moves and practices, exception and routine, and characterized by change as well as continuity over time. This structured empirical analysis can then be used to assess competing normative claims about the ethics and efficacy of securitization as a political strategy. The framework is developed, first, by reimagining securitization as a policy process; and second, by treating the relationship between securitization and desecuritization as a Möbius strip.[1] This framework, by placing change and ongoing meaning-making contests at its analytical core, enables the examination of securitization as a dynamic process unfolding over time. Approaching securitization as a policy process draws attention to variation in the nature and form of meaning-making at different points in the policy cycle, while conceiving of the securitization-desecuritization relationship as a Möbius strip supports consideration of the ways that securitization and desecuritization exist in relationship with each other rather than as binary opposites. In so doing, the framework provides a model for empirical analysis that coherently integrates the study of speech acts, discourse and practice, at multiple levels of analysis and points in space and time, and across several categories of actors. By suggesting sources of persistent limits to the form of meaning-making available within securitization processes, particularly that securitization can only unfold through a reliance on the invocation of threat and consequent establishment of us/Other categories, the framework also supports normative assessment of how and where social justice objectives are best pursued.

To elaborate this framework, the chapter outlines the key propositions of the CS and its sociological and critical interlocutors, and some of their core analytical, empirical and normative debates. It then proposes an integrated framework treating securitization as a contextualized policy process in which speech acts, discourse and practices are equally salient at different points in time, and in which we can see discursive continuities in moments of rupture, and continuity of exceptional practices as issues are partly returned to the realm of normal bureaucratic politics. The chapter concludes by outlining the analytical and methodological implications of the framework, focusing on the method of analysis needed to trace meaning-making contests throughout the securitization process.

The Copenhagen School and its interlocutors[2]

As initially formulated in *Security: A New Framework for Analysis* (Buzan, Wæver, & de Wilde, 1998), the CS defines securitization as a speech act in which an actor in a position of authority identifies an issue as an existential threat. When such a move is successful, this catalyses a break from normal to exceptional securitized politics, thereby justifying rule-breaking and circumvention of normal political processes, especially open, democratic deliberation. "A successful securitization thus has three components (or steps): existential threats, emergency action, and effects on interunit relations by breaking free of rules" (Buzan et al., 1998, p. 26).

The CS framework is premised on three foundational assumptions: that security threats, rather than having a fixed, objective meaning, are established in and through the speech act; that securitizing something makes it a more urgent political priority; and that securitization entails exception, that is, it is through securitization that otherwise unacceptable rule-breaking behaviour, particularly circumvention of debate, deliberation and dialogue, becomes tolerated by virtue of the need to take swift, decisive action against existential threat. The first assumption, that the meaning and content of security is defined through speech acts, was meant to move beyond debates between 'narrow' realist and 'wider', 'deeper' human, critical and feminist security theorists about what security 'really means', and about the appropriate referent object in security discourse and practice. The consequence of privileging speech acts in this way, however, is a core tension in the theory between two explanations of how securitization 'works': the formal linguistics focus on the internal dynamics and structure of the speech act, and the contextually-driven, dynamic process of achieving inter-subjective agreement between securitizing actors and audiences, a process critiqued as "radically underdeveloped" (Williams, 2011, p. 212) in the initial CS framework. This tension has been widely noted (e.g. Balzacq, 2005, 2011; Donnelly, 2013; Stritzel, 2007), and is one that sociological approaches have addressed by foregrounding practices, context and audience-securitizing actor interactions. The other two assumptions are widely shared across otherwise incommensurate theories, including realist, critical, feminist and human security approaches as well as sociological variants of securitization.

The CS's articulation of securitization theory also contains a normative component. While on the one hand stating that theirs is a radically constructivist account in which security has no objective meaning, the CS also maintains a soft normative preference for desecuritization, arguing that "security should be seen as a negative, as a failure to deal with issues as normal politics" (Buzan et al., 1998, p. 29) and that securitization can "[justify] the use of force, the intensification of executive powers, the claim to rights of secrecy, and other extreme measures" (Buzan et al., 1998, p. 208) – suggesting, in other words, that security does objectively entail something undesirable and to be avoided. This normative preference has been more muted in recent CS work, with Wæver (2011, p. 469) now contending that:

> desecuritization is preferable in the abstract but concrete situations might call for securitization.... [T]he "preference" for desecuritization is not of the "political stance" type, but an effect produced by the kinds of analysis that securitization theory spurs: it fosters critical attention to the costs of securitization but allows for the possibility that securitization might help society to deal with important challenges through focusing and mobilizing attention and resources.

Still, while allowing that there may be pragmatic reasons for pursuing securitization in some cases, the CS conception of security remains an essentially negative one, premised on Schmittian exception, elite power and foreclosure of debate (Wæver, 2011, p. 478).

Responses to the CS, which have engaged with both the analytical and normative aspects of securitization theory, can broadly be categorized as 'sociological' and critical.[3] Sociological variants of securitization have first sought to move beyond an exclusive focus on speech acts, arguing that "the political meaning of the security speech act is invested in the notion of 'act' rather than 'speech'" (Huysmans, 2011, p. 372) and that "securitization is better understood as a strategic (pragmatic) process that occurs within, and as part of, a configuration of circumstances.... [S]ecuritization consists of practices which instantiate intersubjective understandings through the habitus inherited from different, often competing social fields" (Balzacq, 2011, pp. 1–2). Consequently, these approaches place greater analytical emphasis on practices, on the context or field within which securitizations occur, and on the active role of the audience in the intersubjective construction of threats (Balzacq, 2005, 2011; Donnelly, 2013; McDonald, 2008; Salter & Piché, 2011; Stritzel, 2007; Williams, 2011). Following from this analytical interest in practices, context and actor-audience dialogue, which necessarily occur over a longer period of time and in several locations, rather than a single moment in time and space (as is the case with an exceptional, securitizing speech act), sociological approaches have a more expansive contextual and temporal focus that troubles the CS's sharp distinction between normal and exceptional politics. For these theorists, acts including mundane technocratic practices, routines and processes (Bigo, 2000, 2001, 2002; Salter & Piché, 2011) and what Huysmans calls "little security nothings" – gradually accruing "unspectacular processes of technologically driven surveillance, risk management and precautionary governance" (Huysmans, 2011, p. 375), which may never produce a moment of exceptional rupture – are what essentially make a securitization.

Critical responses have engaged with the normative aspects of securitization theory in both CS and sociological variants. These responses reflect, and are in many respects a subset of, long-standing debates in the larger field of critical security studies about whether security is an inherently dangerous and negative concept (e.g. Duffield, 2010; Neocleous, 2000, 2008) or holds emancipatory potential (e.g. Booth, 1991; Nunes, 2012; Wyn Jones, 1999). These debates are evident in global health studies (Nunes, 2014; Seckinelgin, 2012), and have also manifested within securitization theory. Here, some interlocutors have developed the initial soft CS preference for desecuritization into a more robust argument about the dangers of securitization and the potential (though also the potential political limits) of desecuritization (Aradau, 2004, 2006; Hansen, 2012), while others have sought to develop securitization as a positive (Floyd, 2007; Roe, 2012) and morally just (Floyd, 2011) concept and political practice. These are not merely normative-theoretical claims; they are also political assertions about the concrete political strategies that ought to be undertaken by those seeking emancipatory and social justice goals, and as such they have important empirical as well as theoretical implications. That is, their prescriptions are not just about what ought normatively to be, but about the empirical efficacy and desirability of securitization and desecuritization as political strategies.

Tensions, limitations and debates

As this brief overview suggests, there remain tensions and debates, as well as some limitations, in securitization theory. These include analytical tensions between CS and sociological perspectives about how security problems are constructed and what, therefore, essentially defines securitization; shared analytical limitations in treatments of history and change in securitization; and third, normative and empirical debates about whether securitization or desecuritization is (a) ethically preferable and (b) functionally more effective at producing emancipatory political change.

CS and sociological variants can certainly be understood as 'ideal types' (Balzacq, 2011) rather than fundamentally incompatible approaches. Indeed, as 'real world' securitizations usually involve multiple elements (e.g. both discourse and practice), empirical studies of securitization often draw on both CS and sociological approaches (Huysmans, 2006; Salter & Mutlu, 2013; Salter & Piché, 2011), notwithstanding that the majority of authors situate themselves closer to one ideal type than the other. Still, there remain important analytical tensions between the two (Balzacq, 2011; Buzan & Hansen, 2009; McDonald, 2008; Stritzel, 2007; Williams, 2011), and these are the subject of lively, ongoing conversations (see for example Gad & Petersen, 2011). One central, unresolved tension revolves around whether securitization requires an exceptional moment, usually in the form of a speech act, constituting a "discontinuous change of state within a social system" (Wæver, 2011, p. 476), or whether securitization can entail an accretion of practices that may not involve a speech act or ever rise to the level of exception (Balzacq, 2011; Huysmans, 2011). This leads to questions about what essentially defines a securitization, and thus how it can be empirically identified and studied. As I discuss below, a policy process model suggests a means of at least partly resolving these tensions, as it shows that these can, instead of being treated as somewhat distinct accounts of how social meaning is created, become two sequential analytical focal points within a single, integrated framework.

Securitization theory also has conceptual limitations when it comes to theorizing change and history. In proposing a discursive approach to norms as processes, Krook and True (2010, p. 106) identify limitations in constructivist treatment of norms that hold equally true for securitization. These include, first, tension between "relatively dynamic accounts of norm [or securitization] creation ... with more static and unitary conceptions of norms [or securitizations] themselves ... [which] limits the ability to explain how and why norms [or securitizations] change as they diffuse". Put differently, the content or meaning of a securitization is often taken as fixed; once the audience is persuaded, there is assumed to be agreement between securitizing actor and audience about why and how a given object, state, etc. constitutes a threat. The meaning of '[X] is a security threat' is then taken to be relatively static over time. But as Krook and True observe, "the acceptance of a norm [or securitization] may initiate rather than resolve struggles over its exact content" (p. 110). Meaning-making contests are ongoing, but the dynamic character of securitization processes, in which meaning is continually made, contested and re-made, can easily be obscured if the content of a securitization is assumed to be stable following a successful securitizing move. To be clear, there is nothing in securitization theory that inherently prevents analysts from identifying change in the meaning of securitizations over time (see for example Donnelly 2013); but neither is there a clear analytical imperative to seek out such change, or a model that would tell us exactly where and how to identify it empirically. Policy process frameworks, in contrast, explicitly theorize and seek out change, suggesting where and how policy interventions (in this case, securitizations) are contested and transformed through the deliberate efforts of policy actors, and how actors themselves revise their perspectives and policies over time.

Securitization theory's difficulties in identifying and theorizing change are exacerbated because it lacks a clear account of securitization as a historical process, and a consistent model for empirical study of this process. For McDonald (2008, p. 576), the problem is that

> long-term processes and practices fit uneasily within the [CS] securitization framework with its focus on "moments" of intervention and the suspension of normal politics ... [and that] focusing on the moment of intervention does not help us understand how or why that particular intervention became possible at that moment. Why then, and in that context, did a particular actor represent an issue as an existential threat, and more importantly why was that actor supported in that securitization by a particular constituency?

As with the treatment of change, there is nothing inherent to securitization theory that would preclude historical analysis, especially in its sociological variants; indeed, there are multiple acknowledgements in the literature that securitization is a historical process (e.g. Balzacq, 2011, p. 14; McDonald, 2008).[4] To further develop and support these inquiries, we require a systematic, structured model, capable of 'travel' across cases; again, policy process models, which approach policy development as an ongoing, iterative process, and propose a means of tracing policies from origins to and outcomes, are capable of supporting precisely this type of empirically-based historical analysis.

Securitization theories are finally characterized by normative debates about the ethics of securitization, which are entangled with empirical assumptions about its efficacy. As already indicated, normative debates centre on two competing claims. One line of argument holds that securitization entails illiberal outcomes and is best avoided in favour of desecuritization, which may itself hold emancipatory potential, while the other suggests that securitization can and should be used to achieve emancipatory ends. With respect to efficacy, CS, sociological and critical variants of securitization all assume and accept that security is the highest political priority, holding unrivalled political power, and thus securitized matters will always trump non-securitized ones. Securitization is therefore assumed to be an effective (if, for some analysts, undesirable) means of attracting attention and resources. Yet this assumption about the power inherent in any invocation of security, while taken as given in much security theory, is actually an empirical proposition to be tested.

A revised framework: securitization as a policy process

Treating securitization as a policy process characterized by ongoing meaning-making contests can, first, provide a means of reconciling some of the tensions and limitations in securitization theory, and, second, offer a framework through which competing functional and normative claims about securitization as a political strategy can be assessed. A policy process framework is not an entirely radical departure from existing approaches: several theorists note in passing that securitization can be considered a political process (Abrahamsen, 2005; Huysmans, 2011; Salter, 2008; Vuori, 2008; Wæver, 2011), and have suggested additional theoretical and analytical approaches that could be joined with securitization theory to accomplish this re-thinking of securitization (Abrahamsen, 2005; Donnelly, 2013; Watson, 2012). Donnelly (2013) suggests that securitization entails iterative, multi-level language games; Salter and Piché (2011, p. 929) describe securitization as "an iterative process within a particular field", while Léonard and Kaunert (2011) draw on Kingdon's policy model and McInnes and Rushton (2013) suggest that securitization be integrated with literature on norm life cycles.

I follow these authors in their sense that *process* needs to be foregrounded in securitization. A policy process approach enables explicit, structured analysis of the historical, bureaucratic and organizational context in which securitizations and subsequent interventions emerge, as well as the way that securitizations are contested and transformed through the deliberate efforts (both discursive and practice-based) of policy actors. That is, a policy process framework can capture dynamism and change as well as continuity, and hold room for a contextualized and historicized approach to speech acts, discourses and practices. It can trace origins, outcomes, meaning-making processes and change at multiple levels and points in time and space.

The most common policy process approach is the basic, parsimonious policy cycle or policy stages model. While numerous variants exist, the basic model as elaborated by Howlett and Ramesh (1995) entails five heuristic categories or stages: *agenda-setting*, comprising the means and mechanisms (including policy windows, policy entrepreneurs (Kingdon, 2003) and discourses (Schmidt, 2008)) through which problems are identified and articulated; *policy formulation*, in which various response options are debated; *decision-making*, in which a course of action is selected; *policy implementation*, in which policy decisions and directives are enacted (and through which initial directives may be re-shaped by political, bureaucratic and other contextual factors (Howlett & Ramesh, 1995, p. 155)); and *policy evaluation and learning*, entailing "an iterative process of active learning on the part of policy actors" (Howlett & Ramesh, 1995, p. 175). The model is not one of linear causality, but a constitutive one in which contests are ongoing and stages may not, empirically, always unfold neatly, discretely and in sequence (Howlett & Ramesh, 1995). Like any model, it entails simplified heuristic categories that enable coherent higher-level analysis of complex empirical processes. But it is precisely this parsimony that facilitates the application of the model to global, IO and other supra-national levels. Below, I propose an adaptation of these policy stages for the study of securitization, elaborating a five-stage model: (1) speech act; (2) framing contest; (3) policy implementation: boundary work; (4) policy implementation: programme development and delivery; and (5) policy learning.

Temporal modification: stages of securitization

The starting point for this framework is the CS insight that securitizing speech acts invoke existential threat to move an issue into the realm of exceptional politics, and that consensus about what constitutes an existential threat is reached intersubjectively. It therefore retains the core elements of the CS criteria for what securitization entails, and treats these as empirical indicators that must be present for us to treat a set of speech acts, policies and practices as a *securitization* policy process. Preserving the centrality of security speech, existential threat and exception addresses a difficulty encountered by sociological approaches that treat securitization as a series of quotidian practices with no identifiable exceptional moment: that this leaves us with no clear, consistent means of identifying securitization. As Williams (2011, p. 218) asks, "If securitization cannot be tied exclusively to extremity and emergency, but comprises a wider spectrum of intensification, including unease and risk … [and] if it is not the word, 'security', nor the breaking free of rules in a spectacular sense, what defines a 'security' act?" By retaining the core CS criteria for securitization (a speech act, invoking existential threat, to justify rule-breaking), albeit as empirical indicators rather than ontological premises, this framework retains a more bounded understanding of securitization than is evident in some sociological approaches, but also provides more consistent guidelines for empirical application.

The retention of these CS criteria for securitization is also a means of placing analytical limits on the framework. Sociological approaches have certainly established the need to consider context, and the literature is filled with passing references to the importance of history; yet if we need to expand the analysis by taking a larger contextual and longer historical view, then we equally need a means of defining this contextual and historical inquiry. McDonald (2008, p. 572), advocating for an expanded approach to securitization, holds that "examining historical 'experiences' with threat designation calls for a looser and highly interpretative approach to analysis which potentially conflicts with the development of a neat and coherent set of 'requirements' to be met for securitization". But without establishing some parameters and requirements, we risk an infinitely open-ended inquiry.

Williams, considering the question of how to identify securitization if neither the word 'security' nor exceptional rule-breaking is present, suggests that a concept of intensification and a focus on fear may be useful. In a sense, the present framework could be understood as a means of understanding securitization as intensification; however, it requires that a securitizing speech act be present, and makes this the analytical starting point. Certainly, once we identify a securitizing speech act, to understand its origins we must start by tracing the history of its emergence. But while this preceding history might be seen as something that intensifies over time, finally culminating in a speech act, this can in the present framework only be identified retroactively. That is, in this framework it is not until after the speech act that we can determine which elements of context and threat discourse to focus on, and tracing discourses of threat (or fear, or unease) if they have not already produced a securitizing speech act does not suffice to show that securitization has occurred.

Retaining the criteria of existential *threat* rather than fear or unease (Williams 2011, Huysmans 2006), also follows CS requirements for securitization. Further, as elaborated in the next chapter, I contend that threat does specific discursive work that fear and unease do not, and that the production of *threatening* objects and subjects is central to securitization. The need for security threats to be posed as *threats*, specifically, has two implications. First, there must be at least partial prior agreement about the meaning and social location of 'threat' for securitizing speech acts to be intelligible and persuasive. This in turn requires us to treat speech acts as a historical production originating in discursive histories that precede, enable and constrain specific speech acts; these speech acts are further shaped by the specific organizational context within which they are articulated. Additionally, once an existential threat has been identified, this implies a need to respond. We therefore need to look beyond the speech act to the practices, i.e. the threat responses, which are produced by it. But securitization's reliance on threat has a second, normative implication, for we can respond to existential threats in only a limited number of ways: we can defend against them, contain them, or aim to eradicate them, but in all cases, an oppositional response is required. This therefore constrains the range of responses possible once an issue has been securitized and therefore placed into the category of existential threat (Wæver, 1995a, pp. 64–65).

The framework also retains the important sociological insight that organizations, especially bureaucracies, are crucial sites for the production and reproduction of security practices over time, and that the professionals who inhabit these sites play just as important a role as elite actors in effecting a securitization. Once we approach securitization as a policy process wherein the speech acts of elite political actors catalyse policy and programmatic effects in bureaucracies, we can treat quotidian practices as a product of securitizing speech acts, and examine the ways that both work in concert and over time to produce securitization of a given issue. We can connect the exceptionality that characterizes securitization – rule-breaking accomplished by invoking urgency and existential threat – to the bureaucratic structures and routines into which that exceptionalism settles over time.

We can also, through policy process models' focus on contestation and change, study these bureaucratic and organizational contexts as sites of debate, dispute, and meaning-making contests. These meaning-making contests vary by their location in the policy process: securitizing speech acts and their discursive antecedents entail contests primarily at the conceptual and discursive level, while the implementation stage is characterized by contests among bureaucratic actors, who engage in boundary work as newly securitized issues and resulting policy directives are incorporated into existing bureaucratic terrain, norms and practice. Meaning-making contests throughout the securitization process occur at different levels and points in time, and entail many different audiences and actors, but in all cases these are characterized by tensions between received categories and efforts to resist or change those categories. At each stage, there is potential for slippage through redefinition of the content and implications of '[X] is a security threat', but at each stage the logic of securitization limits transformative possibilities. In particular, because securitization is precisely meant to exceed the limits of normal politics, fixing meaning in securitization is about the establishment of boundaries, borders and limits. Central questions then become, who is inside or outside of a securitized response? What exceptional transgressions of bodies and territories, in which places, are authorized by securitization? What organizational configurations are required, and especially, who is responsible for leading a securitized response? Meaning-making contests to fix these boundaries occur at discursive, organizational, bodily and territorial levels as we move through the securitization process.

Securitization as a process, then, unfolds as follows (see Figure 2.1). The first stage is a *speech act* invoking existential threat. This modification of the classic policy stages model, in which agenda-setting is the first stage, foregrounds the important role of discourse in threat construction. Crucially, this framework takes the speech act as the analytical but not ontological starting point, and emphasizes that speech acts are historically produced. That is, specific securitizing speech acts become possible because of and are articulated within specific historical contexts, including discursive contexts; thus to understand a securitizing speech act's origins, we must look back in time. Especially, while a given speech act may be provoked by partial rupture or change in the material, discursive or normative context, and may in turn provoke further rupture, there are also continuities at work. In particular, the requirement that security issues must be articulated as existential threats means that an articulation at any given point in time is shaped by prior ideas about threat, particularly ideas about who and what holds potential, even if latent, to be threatening. Therefore, at the first stage of analysis, as we study the speech act itself we must also examine the prior discourses that worked to make the speech act possible: how did longer, historically-produced discourses shape and constrain what could be spoken, how, in this moment? How does this discourse produce a particular configuration of threatened and threatening subjects? We additionally need to consider the material and organizational context of the speech act's emergence, particularly the ways that actors interpret this context. That is, context gives specific form to the expression of larger discourses.

Once a securitizing actor suggests that something is a security threat, this triggers one of many meaning-making contests: debate and contest among elites. This leads to the second stage of securitization, the *framing contest*. In policy stages models, framing is usually collapsed into the first (agenda-setting) policy stage, but in this framework it is proposed as a distinct stage to support finer-grained analysis. At this stage, the contest takes place primarily at the level of words, ideas and language as actors debate the meaning of '[X] is a security threat', especially who or what ought to be understood as threatened and threatening. Often such debates coalesce around simplistic binaries: are immigrants a valued labour source, or a threat to 'our' jobs? Are people with HIV 'innocent

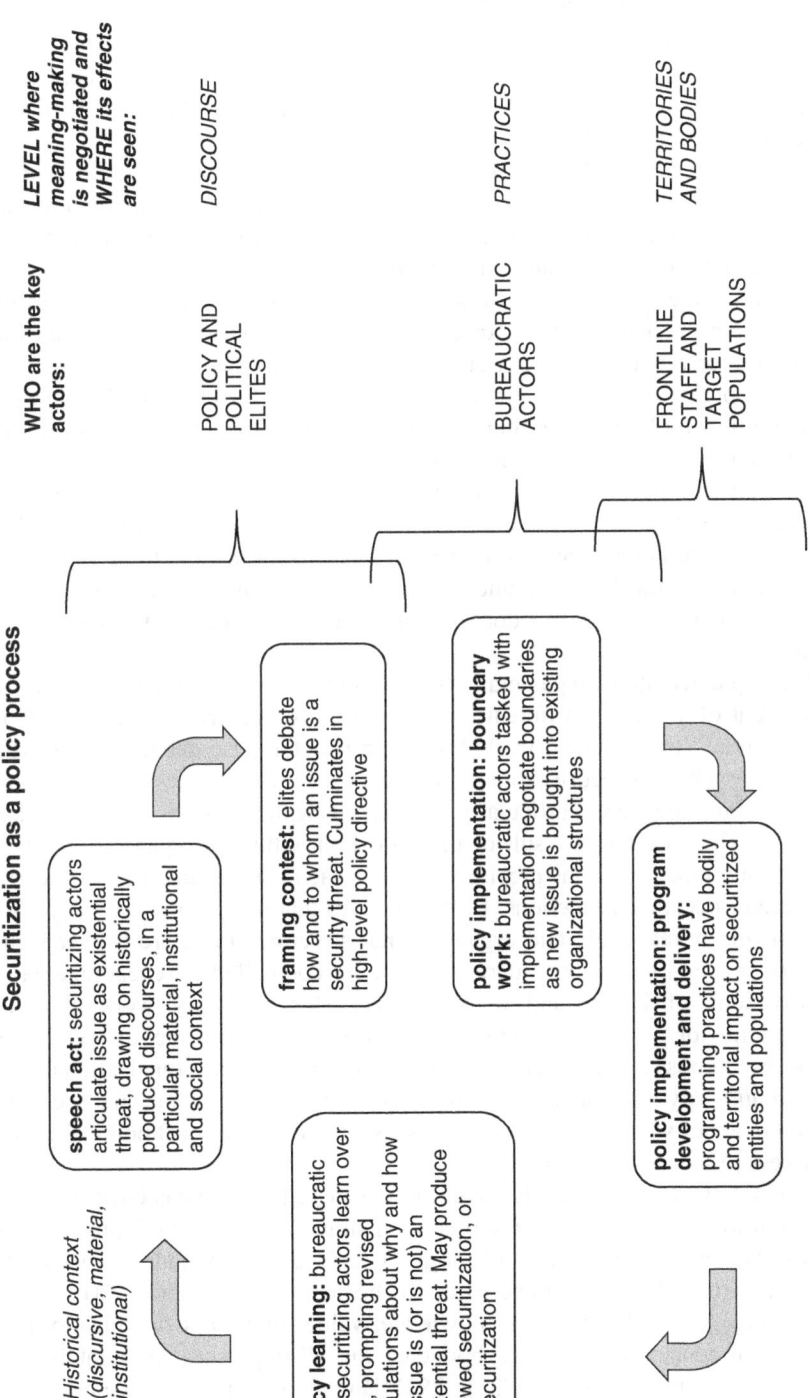

Securitization as a policy process

LEVEL where meaning-making is negotiated and WHERE its effects are seen:

DISCOURSE

PRACTICES

TERRITORIES AND BODIES

WHO are the key actors:

POLICY AND POLITICAL ELITES

BUREAUCRATIC ACTORS

FRONTLINE STAFF AND TARGET POPULATIONS

Historical context (discursive, material, institutional)

speech act: securitizing actors articulate issue as existential threat, drawing on historically produced discourses, in a particular material, institutional and social context

framing contest: elites debate how and to whom an issue is a security threat. Culminates in high-level policy directive

policy implementation: boundary work: bureaucratic actors tasked with implementation negotiate boundaries as new issue is brought into existing organizational structures

policy learning: bureaucratic and securitizing actors learn over time, prompting revised articulations about why and how an issue is (or is not) an existential threat. May produce renewed securitization, or desecuritization

policy implementation: program development and delivery: programming practices have bodily and territorial impact on securitized entities and populations

Figure 2.1 Securitization as a policy process.

victims', or dangerous vectors? Here we see the emergence and solidification of us/Other binaries as securitizing actors draw discursive boundaries between a threatened 'we' who must be defended, and a threatening 'them' or 'it' that is the source of existential threat.

The essence of speech act theory is that by saying words, something is done that exceeds speech. But in the case of securitization, merely achieving intersubjective agreement that something is a threat is insufficient. Speech acts and associated framing contests cannot by themselves meaningfully protect against threat; they merely construct it. A securitizing speech act therefore initiates the securitization process but does not complete it; the discursive move creates an imperative for threat response. Usually, this imperative is conveyed through a high-level policy directive to pursue specific actions, for example the development of policy tools and instruments (Balzacq, 2008; Huysmans, 2006) or border and migration controls (Huysmans, 2006; Salter & Piché, 2011). This catalyses the third stage, where *policy implementation* begins and the process moves from the realm of discourse into the realm of practice, from abstract high-level policy directives to the bureaucratic processes required to implement these directives, and from elite to mid-level bureaucratic actors. As securitization progresses from discourse to practice, so too does our analytic lens shift from discourses to practices.

The implementation stage entails further contests over meaning and categorization, but of a slightly different nature than those occurring at elite levels of policy-making. In particular, while bureaucratic actors also debate exactly what is meant by '[X] is a security threat', and what specific activities threat response should entail, they are particularly concerned with divisions of labour and authority. This is a direct result of their location within an organizational type (bureaucracy) that functions precisely because each component part has clearly-delineated, specialized functions. Elite directives that move a new security issue into existing bureaucratic and organizational structures therefore trigger significant *boundary work* as bureaucratic actors are compelled to renegotiate existing divisions of labour and responsibility. This boundary work also has implications for who is considered to fall within or outside of securitized responses to an issue: bureaucratic actors, as a result of their organizational divisions of authority, may have different understandings than the original securitizing actors about which populations or issues should be the focal point of efforts to address [X] as a security threat.

Boundary work, a sociological concept developed by Thomas Gieryn (1983), is a framework for examining the rhetorical strategies used by scientists to distinguish between 'science' and 'ideology'. Gieryn defines boundary work as the "attribution of selected characteristics to the institution of science (i.e. to its practitioners, methods, stock of knowledge, values and work organization) for purposes of constructing a social boundary that distinguishes some intellectual activities as 'non-science'" (1983, p. 782). Boundary work has since been used by policy scholars writing in interpretive and constructivist traditions "to explain how different disciplines, professions, and social organizations negotiate and maintain the boundaries that delineate their activities and spheres of influence and authority" (Scala, 2007, p. 213). It has primarily been used to examine the negotiation of boundaries between science, technology and politics, but holds potential for much wider use, since it is mainly concerned with illuminating the social construction of different categories of knowledge, professional expertise and spheres of bureaucratic responsibility.

Concurrent with and following from bureaucratic boundary work, the resulting actions or practices to defend against existential threat finally have their ultimate effects on territories and bodies as policies are enacted. At this fourth, *programme development and delivery* stage, our analytical gaze shifts from bureaucratic practices to the material, corporeal terrain of securitized people and things, and from bureaucratic actors to 'on the ground' locales where securitized politics are ultimately played out. Here we can see the ultimate effects of us/ Other binaries and of policy and programming shaped by ideas of 'threat', as we examine who is included in or excluded from securitized responses to a given issue, and the nature of bodily and territorial incursions that are authorized. Additionally, frontline staff may have yet another interpretation, different from both securitizing and bureaucratic actors, about who and what is or is not implicated in '[X] is a security threat'; thus meaning-making and categorization contests are also evident at this stage. Practices and bureaucracies remain important here, too: over time we see a gradual routinization of this work as securitized responses partially settle into the realm of mid-level bureaucratic rather than elite political responsibility. That is, the processes through which a securitized response unfolds are at least partly bureaucratic in nature, and necessarily entail a partial settling in the structures that also support everyday practices of desecuritized politics.

There is a further stage of securitization as practices and programmes unfold over time. Especially where an issue had not previously been identified as a security threat, policy implementation produces a new field of policy, programming (and often academic) expertise. Following initial boundary work to determine who should have responsibility for the new programming area of '[X] and/ in security', bureaucratic actors then must establish themselves as a source of technical or expert authority on the matter; again, this is the logical consequence of imperatives inherent to bureaucracy as an organizational form. Actors gradually redefine and resituate themselves as experts in the securitized response to [X], and observe the consequences of their work (both on the ground and within their bureaucracy or organization). Through these observations and the accrual of expert technical knowledge, both they and initial securitizing actors learn over time.

This *actor learning* is the fifth stage of the securitization process. While traditional policy stages models often propose policy evaluation as the fifth stage, the present framework follows elaborations of the model that expand 'evaluation' to broadly encompass actor learning (Howlett & Ramesh, 1995). For securitizations, which often entail exception and circumvention of structured, formal processes such as outcome evaluation, an expansive stage of actor learning that can also encompass informal or experiential learning is more appropriate than a tightly bounded formal policy evaluation stage.

As actors learn what securitization can do for them (e.g. give them greater autonomy, resources or authority), or as they identify limitations in the initial securitization that they wish to rectify, they may seek a return to an earlier, urgently securitized state via a re-statement of the original speech act, '[X] is a security threat', by elite securitizing actors in structurally powerful positions. Yet this re-statement may, because of what actors have learned, entail a different articulation of how and to whom [X] is a threat. If successful, this brings us full circle, back to meaning-making contests at the level of elite political discourse. If unsuccessful, or if actors eventually cease to regard an issue as an existential threat, it may settle further into bureaucratic politics, gradually becoming desecuritized as once-exceptional practices become a matter of routine. Here too there are continuities: the exceptional practices that were initially justified through the invocation of existential threat become 'everyday exceptions', often expanding and deepening over time as bureaucratic actors, now constituted as experts on this policy matter, exercise autonomy and pursue programming directions different to those originally envisioned by securitizing actors.

This feature of securitization and desecuritization – that the deepest bodily and territorial incursions do not necessarily emerge at the initial, acute securitized moment, but rather may emerge years later, through bureaucratic practices much closer to normal than securitized politics – provides the impetus for a second theoretical move: reimagining the relationship between securitization and desecuritization.

Conceptual modification: de/securitization as Möbius strip

Once we approach securitization as a policy process unfolding over time, we can find significant continuities between securitized and desecuritized politics. There are, first, discursive continuities at work as an issue is moved, via a speech act relying on prior ideas about threat, into the realm of exceptional securitized politics. Second, at the other end of the securitization process, an issue that has become at least partially desecuritized as it settles into routine bureaucratic procedures may still entail programming responses that are exceptional and rule-breaking in nature. Securitization and desecuritization bleed into each other. There is especially no clear dividing line, no instant where we can say that an issue decisively and completely moves from securitized into desecuritized politics (it seems to be a more gradual process, identifiable in retrospect but resulting from gradual discursive and material shifts over time, not one decisive move in a single moment), but neither is the initial move into securitized politics a complete break from normal politics.

Therefore, this framework conceptualizes securitization and desecuritization not as binary opposites, but as a Möbius strip. A Möbius strip has only one surface; inside and outside are collapsed into a single plane. It is conceptually useful for thinking about securitization and desecuritization as relational processes, and for attending to the continuities that exist throughout the securitization process. That is, rather than representing a moment of complete rupture and separation from normal politics, a Möbius formation helps us think of securitizations as historically produced, and entailing some continuities that run through normal, securitized and desecuritized politics. Pragmatically, approaching securitization as an iterative process helps us draw analytical links between acute points of securitization (identifiable through speech acts) and seemingly unexceptional phenomena (usually involving practices) more temporally and spatially distant from securitizing speech. This furthermore reminds us that desecuritization does not preclude exception: rupture and rule-breaking are not restricted to a single securitized moment, and while it may be easier to justify a greater range of exceptional practices at the initial point at which an issue is successfully positioned as an existential threat, these are not necessarily stopped or undone as issues return, over time, to the realm of desecuritized politics.

If there are exceptional practices in desecuritized politics and if securitization itself is produced in part through continuities originating in normal politics, why should we consider one state as preferable to the other, or as holding greater potential for emancipatory change? The answer is that this framework retains the CS insight that securitization is triggered by the invocation of 'threat' – this is what moves an issue into the security field, and it is ideas about 'threat' that subsequently inform the logic and practice of securitization. No such constraints need exist in normal politics, meaning that a wider range of options exist in normal politics than exist once an issue is securitized. While exceptional practices can and often do continue into desecuritized politics, they do not *have* to; but such practices, considered a necessary part of threat response, are an inherent, defining feature of securitization. Further, even the exceptions that continue into desecuritized politics are originally made possible through the logic of securitization and its invocation of threat. My point in drawing attention to the continuities between securitized and desecuritized moments in the policy process is merely that we cannot be sanguine about the return of an issue to desecuritized politics, nor should we assume that this is sufficient to protect against exception. Consequently, the question 'desecuritization into what' warrants close attention. We also need to remember that this Möbius strip is not a model of the whole of normal politics, but of the relationship between securitized and desecuritized politics. Outside of and beyond the realm of desecuritization (which implies a prior securitization – only that which has been securitized can be *de*securitized) is a universe of normal politics encompassing issues that have never been brought into the security field, and forms of politics not predicated on threat construction and response.

Others positing securitization as a process have suggested treating securitization as a continuum (Abrahamsen, 2005; McInnes & Rushton, 2013), but this still, at either extreme, implies binaries. A Möbius formation instead requires us to see securitization and desecuritization as always relational and entangled. While there may be analytical use in treating the two as ideal types, in practical politics there is no 'pure' securitized or desecuritized state. Rather, exceptions follow us into desecuritized politics, and discursive treatment of some things as 'threatening' precedes, enables and continues into exceptional securitized politics. The great advantage to thinking about securitization and desecuritization as existing on a Möbius strip is then that it avoids perpetuating binary either/or categories and strong heuristic divisions, allowing us to study securitization and desecuritization as relational and disrupting the assumption of binary states (us/ Other; exceptional/normal; securitized/desecuritized; inside/outside) upon which both empirical securitizing moves and much securitization theory are predicated.

This conceptual modification then facilitates assessment of functional and normative claims about securitization as a political strategy, particularly by drawing attention to the ways that securitizing speech acts are inherently bounded by historically-produced threat discourses. While there is contestation throughout the securitization process, these contests rely on ideas about 'threat' that produce and reinforce binary us/Other and threatened/threatening divisions. This has profound normative and ethical consequences, as it limits the terrain of debate and action to that which is permissible within the logic of securitization. The contest within this logic consists of deciding where the line between us and Other is to be drawn, rather than asking how or if this line might be erased. Even where securitization is undertaken in support of transformative political strategies, once an issue is positioned as an existential threat it is this logic that prevails. Subsequently, because the logic and meaning-making processes of securitization produce exclusion by defining boundaries and limits, there would seem to be little room for emancipatory or solidarity-based politics within a securitized response. Of course, this proposition requires empirical assessment, but it is presented here to indicate how the analytical framework supports the normative argument developed through the rest of the book.

Analytical and methodological implications

There are analytical implications to approaching securitization as a policy process in which there is an iterative relationship between discourse and its material effects, and in which securitization and desecuritization are related and entail continuities as well as disruption. Essentially, at different points in the policy process, there are different analytical focal points. This means that when studying empirical cases of securitization, we need a process and set of analytical tools that allow us to, from a speech act, work back in time and up in levels of abstraction to discover its origins, and forward in time and downward in level of abstraction to trace the speech act's effects – including effects that may be quite temporally removed from initial securitizing speech and may at first seem to be desecuritized everyday practices, but that on closer examination contain within them the exceptions and excesses of securitization. We need, that is, a way to discover and describe relationships between *articulated ideas*; the *actions or practices* that follow from them, as well as the *material effects* of these actions; the *underlying assumptions* required for these ideas and actions to make sense, and the *discourses* that shape or inform these assumptions; and the *material and organizational conditions* that shape the speech act's emergence. Because this is an iterative process, we also need to consider *actor learning* and how this produces changes in the content of securitizations over time (see Figure 2.2).

The analytical starting point is the articulated ideas that comprise the securitizing speech act. We begin with articulated ideas because these can be traced and triangulated, as can subsequent actions (including efforts to persuade others, policy development and implementation, and bureaucratic boundary work) and material effects that follow from these ideas and actions. The speech act, that is, serves as an identifiable moment of articulation that tells us a securitizing move is occurring. However, the ontological work of making securitization possible has already occurred by the time the speech act is articulated, and material effects cannot be foretold from speech alone. To understand the origins and effects of securitization we must look before the speech act (to historical processes that make some things but not others thinkable as threats, to securitizing actors' encounters with these threats, and to the discourses through which these

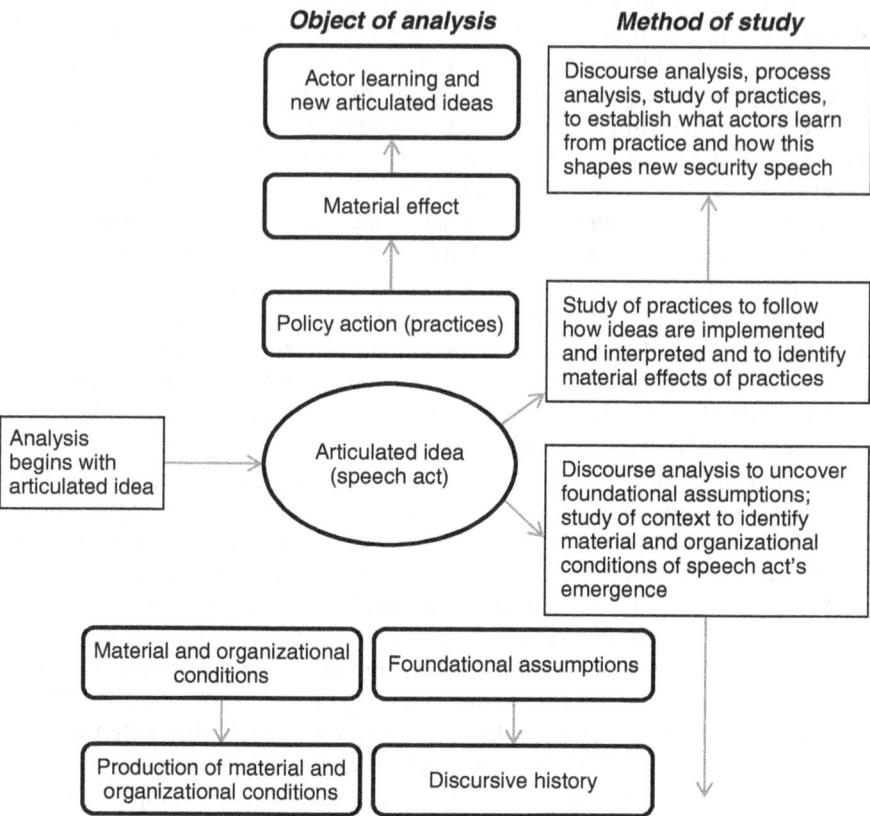

Figure 2.2 Analytical approach.

encounters are mediated) and after speech (to discursive, policy, programming and bodily effects).

Therefore, after identifying the articulated ideas in the speech act, we ask: For this articulated idea to make sense, what foundational assumptions are required? Once foundational assumptions are uncovered, we can discover how a given securitization became 'thinkable' in the first place by tracing how larger, longer discourses worked over time to produce these foundational assumptions. I have termed this the 'discursive history' of the speech act. The discursive focus here does not imply that the material context is unimportant: "[t]he point is not to disregard material facts but to study how these are produced and prioritized" (Hansen, 2006, p. 20). Establishing any entity's status as threatening entails a discursive process of interpreting material realities, and it is this discursive production that makes a securitization thinkable and speakable. The aim, then, is to understand at a discursive level how and why a given speech act takes the form that it does: what historically-produced discourses made it thinkable and speakable in that particular way? Importantly, this analysis can only ever be retroactive: we do not know which aspects of discourse to study until after the speech act, which is the point at which we can say with certainty that a securitization is occurring. Only then can we untangle the discursive antecedents that do the ontological work of threat construction in a given instance from the infinite other discourses that could potentially become part of a securitization.[5]

We must also examine the proximate context of the speech act's emergence, i.e. the organizational, material and other contextual factors that shape the precise content and form of articulations about threat. This likewise entails working backwards from the speech act to identify experiences, practices, and aspects of the material or organizational context – and, crucially, the ways that these are interpreted by actors – either explicitly identified by securitizing actors as having influenced their decision to securitize, or that can be reasonably understood as having influenced that decision. The present study mainly draws on interviews, and textual and organizational analysis, but a diverse range of interpretive methods could be used to explore the larger context in which the speech act emerges and framing contests occur.

To understand the consequences of securitization, we also need to identify the practices and material effects it produces. This entails process analysis and the study of practices to identify the impact of securitizing speech acts (articulated ideas) on bureaucratic practices, 'on the ground' programming, and on bodies and territories. Finally, to understand the evolution of securitization over time, we return to securitizing actors to examine what they have learned through the policy implementation process. Here, both practices and discourses are studied to explore how actors revise their understanding of how and why a given issue is a security threat based on what they have learned through observing the policy implementation process and its effects. The present study has mainly used interviews, textual analysis and process analysis to uncover policy impact and actor learning, but depending on the nature of the empirical case under investigation, a wide range of ethnographic and other interpretive methods might be appropriate.

Conclusion

This chapter has proposed treating securitization as a policy process in which meaning-making contests are ongoing, but occurring at different levels (discourse, bureaucratic practices, bodies and territories) and involving different actors and audiences (political elites, mid-level bureaucrats, frontline staff and target populations) at different stages of the policy process (speech act, policy framing, implementation, programme delivery and actor learning over time). The framework does not, of course, fully resolve all tensions and debates in securitization theory: those who contend that securitization does not require a speech act, or the crossing of some threshold of extremity, will remain unsatisfied with the retention of these as empirical criteria for securitization. It additionally, by retaining the requirement that a speech act be present, remains only partly able to address silence as an expression of insecurity (Hansen, 2000), in that silences would need to be understood as the effect of securitizing speech and action that renders silent subjects insecure, and/or as part of the conditions of the speech act's emergence. Similarly, the retention of the speech act means that images (Williams, 2003) cannot, by themselves, be understood as sufficient to constitute a securitization, though they certainly may be part of the context that makes securitizing speech acts 'thinkable'.

Yet the framework can productively advance securitization theory. It treats CS and sociological approaches' respective privileging of speech acts or contextual factors (practices, actor-audience interactions, etc.) not as theoretical commitments made by the analyst prior to empirical inquiry, but as sequential analytical focal points that are each equally salient at different points in the policy process. This supports coherent integration of several strands of securitization theory into a single analytical framework for structured empirical inquiry. Further, because the framework uses a basic policy process model, it would likely travel well to other scales and sites of analysis, and could equally be applied to micro and macrosecuritizations (Buzan & Wæver, 2009) as well as the 'middle level' securitizations that were the initial focus of the framework (Buzan et al., 1998). That is, policy and ensuing practices are not produced solely by states, but can also be produced at the global level by IOs (as in this study), by sub-national entities including municipalities and neighbourhood associations, by NGOs, or by firms. Treating securitization as a policy process therefore provides us with a framework through which even micro-level securitizations, or those undertaken by non-state actors, can be recognized and analysed.

In sum, a policy process model integrates multiple levels of analysis, categories of actors, sites of securitizing speech and practice, and stages of policymaking in a single framework that supports the systematic analysis of the emergence, evolution and effects of securitization. This analysis then supports subsequent normative assessment of the potential for securitization, as a political strategy, to support social justice projects and produce emancipatory change. The rest of the book uses this framework (and the analytical process it implies) to explore the case of HIV securitization, and to develop some of the theoretical claims introduced in this chapter.

Notes

1 Bigo (2001) uses the Möbius ribbon to describe the collapsing of internal and external security practices into a single securitization regime. While he uses the Möbius ribbon to make the empirical argument that there is no longer a meaningful functional distinction between police and military security practices, I use it to make a conceptual argument about the relationship between securitization and desecuritization.

2 While there are limitations in 'schools' designations (see for example the c.a.s.e. collective 2006), use of 'Copenhagen School' to denote the originators of securitization theory, particularly Ole Wæver and Barry Buzan, follows what is by now well-established convention in the literature. Similarly, I follow a core text (Balzacq, 2011) in using the term 'sociological' to refer to Bourdieusian- and Foucauldian-inspired variants of securitization that emphasize performativity, practices, and actor-audience dynamics. Like any categories, these are heuristic and meant to support structured analysis. Use of the term 'critical' to denote the broad category of literature engaging with normative aspects of securitization theory is less common, but reflects that these engagements share, with all critical projects, concern for not only what is, but what ought to be; that is, they have prescriptive and transformative objectives (largely, though not exclusively, pertaining to emancipation).

3 This section presents a brief summary of some of the core debates in, and with, CS, with a view towards drawing out the main analytical, empirical and normative problematiques with which this book engages. For further discussion of sociological critiques of CS, see for example Buzan and Hansen (2009), Balzacq (2011) and Williams (2011). For assessments of the critical security studies project (both of which situate the CS within critical security studies, although the CS itself clearly distinguishes securitization theory from CSS), see for example Browning and McDonald (2011) and Hynek and Chandler (2013).

4 Most empirical studies of securitization focus on contemporary practices (e.g. Bigo, 2002; Salter & Piché, 2011), but for historical analysis see for example Stritzel (2012) or Salter and Mutlu (2013). Wæver has elaborated a discursive approach to conceptual history in his studies of European security (1995a, 1995b, 1996) and the evolution of ideas about peace and security (2008). A conceptual history approach is in tension with the CS framework wherein the speech act itself, not its longer historical antecedents, creates a given securitization. This may explain why, as Wæver acknowledges (2000, p. 251), his policy-focused analyses of European security, identity and peace research, in which he most clearly articulates a conceptual history approach, have proceeded somewhat separately from his securitization research agenda with/in the CS.

5 The definition of 'discourse' is intentionally left open, as the aim is to introduce an analytical framework that could be used by analysts with a range of theoretical and methodological commitments, including different understandings of discourse, to study empirical instances of securitization. Chapter 3 provides a definition of how discourse is understood in this book.

References

Abrahamsen, R. (2005). Blair's Africa: The politics of securitization and fear. *Alternatives*, *30*(1), 55–80.

Aradau, C. (2004). Security and the democratic scene: desecuritization and emancipation. *Journal of International Relations and Development*, *7*(4), 388–413.

Aradau, C. (2006). Limits of security, limits of politics? A response. *Journal of International Relations and Development, 9*(1), 81–90.

Balzacq, T. (2005). The three faces of securitization: political agency, audience and context. *European Journal of International Relations, 11*(2), 171–201.

Balzacq, T. (2008). The policy tools of securitization: information exchange, EU foreign and interior policies. *Journal of Common Market Studies, 46*(1), 75–100.

Balzacq, T. (2011). A theory of securitization: origins, core assumptions, variants. In T. Balzacq (Ed.), *Securitization Theory: How Security Problems Emerge and Dissolve* (pp. 1–30). New York: Routledge.

Bigo, D. (2000). When two become one: internal and external securitisations in Europe. In M. Kelstrup & M. C. Williams (Eds.), *International Relations Theory and the Politics of European Integration: Power, Security and Community* (pp. 171–204). New York: Routledge.

Bigo, D. (2001). The Möbius ribbon of internal and external security(ies). In M. Albert, D. Jacobson, & Y. Lapid (Eds.), *Identities, Borders, Orders: Rethinking International Relations Theory* (pp. 91–116). Minneapolis, MN: University of Minnesota Press.

Bigo, D. (2002). Security and Immigration: toward a critique of the governmentality of unease. *Alternatives: Global, Local, Political, 27*(1), 63–92.

Booth, K. (1991). Security and emancipation. *Review of International Studies, 17*(4), 313–326.

Browning, C. S. & McDonald, M. (2011). The future of critical security studies: ethics and the politics of security. *European Journal of International Relations, 19*(2), 235–255.

Buzan, B. & Hansen, L. (2009). *The Evolution of International Security Studies*. Cambridge, UK: Cambridge University Press.

Buzan, B. & Wæver, O. (2009). Macrosecuritisation and security constellations: reconsidering scale in securitization theory. *Review of International Studies, 35*(2), 253–276.

Buzan, B., Wæver, O., & de Wilde, J. (1998). *Security: A New Framework for Analysis*. Boulder, CO: Lynne Rienner.

c.a.s.e. collective. (2006). Critical approaches to security in Europe: a networked manifesto. *Security Dialogue, 37*(4), 443–487.

Donnelly, F. (2013). *Securitization and the Iraq War: The Rules of Engagement in World Politics*. New York: Routledge.

Duffield, M. (2010). The liberal way of development and the development–security impasse: exploring the global life–chance divide. *Security Dialogue, 41*(1), 53–76.

Floyd, R. (2007). Towards a consequentialist evaluation of security: bringing together the Copenhagen and the Welsh schools of security studies. *Review of International Studies*, (33), 327–350.

Floyd, R. (2011). Can securitization theory be used in normative analysis? Towards a just securitization theory. *Security Dialogue, 42*(4–5), 427–439.

Gad, U. P. & Petersen, K. L. (Eds.) (2011). Special issue on the politics of securitization. *Security Dialogue, 42*(4–5), 315–480.

Gieryn, T. F. (1983). Boundary-work and the demarcation of science from non-science: strains and interests in professional ideologies of scientists. *American Sociological Review, 48*(6), 781–795.

Hansen, L. (2000). The Little Mermaid's silent security dilemma and the absence of gender in the Copenhagen School. *Millennium: Journal of International Studies, 29*(2), 285–306.

Hansen, L. (2006). *Security As Practice: Discourse Analysis and the Bosnian War*. New York: Routledge.

Hansen, L. (2012). Reconstructing desecuritization: the normative-political in the Copenhagen School and directions for how to apply it. *Review of International Studies, 38,* 525–546.

Howlett, M. & Ramesh, M. (1995). *Studying Public Policy: Policy Cyles and Policy Subsytems.* Toronto: Oxford University Press.

Huysmans, J. (2006). *The Politics of Insecurity: Fear, Migration and Asylum in the EU.* New York: Routledge.

Huysmans, J. (2011). What's in an act? On security speech acts and little security nothings. *Security Dialogue, 45*(4–5), 371–383.

Hynek, N. & Chandler, D. (2013). No emancipatory alternative, no critical security studies. *Critical Studies on Security, 1*(1), 46–63.

Kingdon, J. W. (2003). *Agendas, Alternatives and Public Policies* (2nd edn). New York: Longman.

Krook, M. L. & True, J. (2010). Rethinking the life cycles of international norms: the United Nations and the global promotion of gender equality. *European Journal of International Relations, 18*(1), 103–127.

Léonard, S. & Kaunert, C. (2011). Reconceptualizing the audience in securitization theory. In T. Balzacq (Ed.), *Securitization Theory: How Security Problems Emerge and Dissolve* (pp. 57–76). New York: Routledge.

McDonald, M. (2008). Securitization and the construction of security. *European Journal of International Relations, 14*(4), 563–587.

McInnes, C. & Rushton, S. (2013). HIV/AIDS and securitization theory. *European Journal of International Relations, 19*(1), 115–138.

Neocleous, M. (2000). Against security. *Radical Philosophy, 100*(2), 7–15.

Neocleous, M. (2008). *Critique of Security.* Montreal: McGill-Queen's University Press.

Nunes, J. (2012). Reclaiming the political: emancipation and critique in security studies. *Security Dialogue, 43*(4), 345–361.

Nunes, J. (2014). *Security, Emancipation and the Politics of Health: A New Theoretical Perspective.* New York: Routledge.

Roe, P. (2012). Is securitization a 'negative' concept? Revisiting the normative debate over normal versus extraordinary politics. *Security Dialogue, 43*(3), 249–266.

Salter, M. B. (2008). Securitization and desecuritization: a dramaturgical analysis of the Canadian Air Transport Security Authority. *Journal of International Relations and Development, 11*(4), 321–349.

Salter, M. B. & Mutlu, C. E. (2013). Securitisation and Diego Garcia. *Review of International Studies, 39*(4), 815–834.

Salter, M. B. & Piché, G. (2011). The securitization of the US–Canada border in American political discourse. *Canadian Journal of Political Science, 44*(4), 929–951.

Scala, F. (2007). Scientists, government and "boundary work": the case of reproductive technologies and genetic engineering in Canada. In M. Orsini & M. Smith (Eds.), *Critical Policy Studies* (pp. 211–231). Vancouver: UBC Press.

Schmidt, V. A. (2008). Discursive institutionalism: the explanatory power of ideas and discourse. *Annual Review of Political Science, 11*, 303–326.

Seckinelgin, H. (2012). *International Security, Conflict and Gender: "HIV/AIDS is Another War".* New York: Routledge.

Stritzel, H. (2007). Towards a theory of securitization: Copenhagen and beyond. *European Journal of International Relations, 13*(3), 357–383.

Stritzel, H. (2012). Securitization, power, intertextuality: discourse theory and the translations of organized crime. *Security Dialogue, 43*(6), 549–567.

Vuori, J. A. (2008). Illocutionary logic and strands of securitisation – applying the theory of securitisation to the study of non-democratic political orders. *European Journal of International Relations, 14*(1), 65–99.

Wæver, O. (1995a). Securitization and desecuritization. In R. D. Lipschutz (Ed.), *On Security* (pp. 46–86). New York: Columbia University Press.

Wæver, O. (1995b). Identity, integration and security: solving the sovereignty puzzle in E.U. studies. *Journal of International Affairs, 48*(2), 389–431.

Wæver, O. (1996). European security identities. *Journal of Common Market Studies, 34*(1), 103–132.

Wæver, O. (2000). The EU as a security actor: reflections from a pessimistic constructivist on post-sovereign security orders. In M. Kelstrup & M. C. Williams (Eds.), *International Relations Theory and the Politics of European Integration: Power, Security and Community* (pp. 250–294). New York: Routledge.

Wæver, O. (2008). Peace and security: two evolving concepts and their changing relationship. In H. G. Brauch, N. C. Behera, B. Chourou, P. Dunay, J. Grin, P. Mbote-Kameri, P. H. Liotta, C. Mesjasz, & U. O. Spring (Eds.), *Globalization and Environmental Challenges: Reconceptualizing Security in the 21st Century* (pp. 99–112). Berlin: Springer.

Wæver, O. (2011). Politics, security, theory. *Security Dialogue, 42*(4–5), 465–480.

Watson, S. D. (2012). 'Framing' the Copenhagen School: integrating the literature on threat construction. *Millennium: Journal of International Studies, 40*(2), 279–301.

Williams, M. C. (2003). Words, images, enemies: securitization and international politics. *International Studies Quarterly, 47*(4), 511–531.

Williams, M. C. (2011). The continuing evolution of securitization theory. In T. Balzacq (Ed.), *Securitization Theory: How Security Problems Emerge and Dissolve* (pp. 212–222). New York: Routledge.

Wyn Jones, R. (1999). *Security, Strategy and Critical Theory*. Boulder, CO: Lynne Rienner.

3 Africa, HIV and security

The discursive context of threat construction in securitization

The previous chapter introduced two claims about how securitization works. First, securitization relies on the invocation of *threat*. This means that we need to examine historically produced discourses – which I have called discursive histories – that work over time to make some things thinkable and then speakable as threats. Second, the organizational context of the speech act significantly influences exactly how these articulations can be spoken and recognized as legitimate security speech. Therefore, to understand the origins and form of securitizing speech, a dual inquiry is needed: into the macro-level discourses working over an extended time to produce subjects, issues, etc. as threatening, and into the production of security meaning and practice in the specific organizational context of the speech act. In both cases, this inquiry entails working backwards from empirically-identifiable aspects of the speech act to discover the conditions in and through which invocations of existential threat become possible, as well as the constraints inherent in those conditions.

This chapter, then, sets the stage for analysis of HIV securitization by working backwards from two empirical observations about the securitizing speech acts made in the UNSC sessions in 2000: the initial speech acts positioned HIV as a specifically *African* threat, and they used national and human security language to do so. Our analytical aim is to discover the discursive histories that made HIV thinkable as a security threat, with particular reference to Africa, and in a manner consistent with national and human security; and to discover how the UN's institutionalized definitions of security in and through which these claims were articulated worked to shape the parameters of intelligible security speech. This is neither a teleological argument about the inevitability of HIV securitization, nor a causal argument about *why* HIV was securitized. It is a constitutive argument, an inquiry into the conditions of possibility in which HIV as a security threat could become thinkable and speakable, and the constraints inherent in those conditions of possibility. While the deliberate efforts of securitizing actors were one proximate cause of the UNSC sessions, and are considered in the next chapter, to understand the origins of this speech act we must first uncover how claims about HIV, Africa and security made during the sessions could have become thinkable in the first place.

The argument is that HIV as a security threat became thinkable (in both national and human security terms) because HIV was *already* generally held to be threatening, particularly because of its association with specific populations and regions. In particular, HIV was already associated with Africa, and Africa in turn was already produced as a threatening Other through racialized discourses associating Africa with disorder, violent conflict and non-normative states and sexuality, all of which worked to produce difference and hierarchy. Thus 'threat' worked at a macro level to unite discourses about HIV, Africa and security, and made 'HIV is a security threat' thinkable in particular ways. Conditions of possibility were further shaped at the organizational level, where national and human security provide the already-agreed upon meanings of security in the UN system, which already placed limits on the ways that HIV could be securitized in that system. Additionally, 'security' in the UN system is the remit of specific actors in specific locations, which additionally constrains how and by whom security can be spoken. These macro-discursive and local organizational contexts worked together to shape the parameters and contours – the conditions and limits of discursive possibility – within which HIV became thinkable as a security threat.

The chapter begins by clarifying what is meant by discourse and why a discursive approach is needed to illuminate how material conditions are interpreted. It then elaborates on the centrality of threat construction in securitization, and therefore the importance of tracing how threat and security are discursively produced, both historically and organizationally. The chapter then turns to the discursive history of HIV, Africa and threat construction, showing how Africa and HIV become differently thinkable in these discourses as threatened (in human security) or threatening (in national security) terms – but also that emancipatory and transformative discourses have tended to operate entirely outside the logic of threat construction, making such claims more difficult to articulate even in the ostensibly capacious language of human security. The subsequent section explores how human and national security work – in terms of their internal logic, and in the context of the UN system – to limit what can be spoken as a threat, where, and by whom. The chapter concludes with a reflection on the implications that the production of these discursively- and organizationally-defined limits have for securitization.

Discourse and materiality in HIV securitization

Sceptical readers may ask whether the focus on discourse is not misplaced. After all, HIV was undoubtedly having a materially devastating impact in the form of high prevalence rates and AIDS deaths, especially in sub-Saharan Africa; and technological progress in the form of ARVs had materially contributed to the surge in activism, in the late 1990s and early 2000s, for improved treatment access. Certainly HIV securitization was in part a response to these material conditions. Yet the rationalization that 'of course' HIV was an existential threat for self-evident material reasons itself suggests just how deeply we are conditioned to think of 'threat' as applying to some things and not others, and to naturalize this as 'objectively material' without considering how discourse might be working to mediate our interpretation of that materiality. This becomes evident if we consider that, first, rates of HIV in 2000 were also high in several non-African states (Joint United Nations Programme on HIV/AIDS (UNAIDS), 2008) whose pandemics nevertheless were not securitized by the UNSC. Additionally, in Africa and elsewhere, several other diseases kill more people annually than HIV, and might arguably have constituted a more immediate threat and urgent priority than HIV; these include diarrheal disease, which spreads more easily and rapidly than HIV, and kills a greater number of people annually (United Nations Children's Fund (UNICEF) & World Health Organization (WHO), 2009). Yet it was HIV, not some other disease, with initial reference to Africa, not some other region, which was securitized. This does not mean the material does not 'matter', but it suggests reasons beyond brute materiality for HIV securitization.

Put differently, the status of HIV and/in Africa as a *threat* is a discursive production that entails interpretation, not objective representation, of material realities. HIV was having (and continues to have) a devastating impact on sub-Saharan countries and communities, but there is no inherent reason why this should be understood in terms of threat and security. The pandemic required (and continues to require) sustained attention and resource allocation, but this could be framed as a matter of social justice, equity, or a moral imperative, rather than a security threat. We therefore require a discursive explanation to understand how these material phenomena could be interpreted specifically as *threats* in need of securitization.

All of this requires us to ask how discourses, particularly discourses about Africa, HIV and security, could have worked to render thinkable the threat constructions inherent to securitization. To uncover the complex dynamics at work in the construction of threatening subjects, an expansive definition of discourse is warranted. Following Foucault's archaeological approach (2002 [1970]), discourses are defined here as ordering modes of thought that underlie systems of classification and categorization, and that shape, often unconsciously, our perception of the world. Discourses operate at a high level of abstraction and at the level of the social environment, beyond and before individual actors' cognitive processes, thought and speech. Discourses form the context within and through which ideas are established and expressed; that is, discourses create the conditions of possibility within which ideas become possible, or 'thinkable'. They do so in subtle and complex ways, by suggesting which aspects of the social landscape are most significant, and how to understand relationships between diverse objects, concepts, populations and territories. In the case of HIV securitization, our primary aim is to discover how discourses established relationships between HIV, Africa and security, especially via overlapping categories of threat, thereby rendering them susceptible to securitization.

The centrality of threat in securitization

While a foundational concept to almost all security theory and practice, the concept of threat, per se, has received surprisingly little attention; in many respects we have talked around it, couching discussions about threat in larger discussions about the meaning of security (Huysmans, 1998, 2006; Mathews, 1989; McDonald, 2002, 2008; Rothschild, 1995; Ullman, 1983). Yet the two concepts are not interchangeable. For incisive empirical analysis, we need to understand the role that threat, specifically, plays in securitization.

Securitization evokes a specific type of urgency and political response by invoking existential *threat*. Threat designation implies not just an inside/outside distinction, but also that what is outside is both different from and threatening to those designated as inside (Aradau, 2004; Huysmans, 2006). The invocation of threat, that is, designates an Other that is set apart from and rendered less valuable than the threatened referent object. It is a normative as well as a categorical judgement, and it produces not just difference but hierarchy and antagonistic relations (Huysmans, 2006) based on that difference. Threat construction produces relations with little room for nuance, complexity or rapprochement between us and Other, and this in turn implies a limited range of responses: in the logic of securitization, threat response can only be oppositional. Empirically, this typically entails policies and programmes designed with the primary aim of containment, control, eradication or other defensive or protective measures to guard against a dangerous Other (Davies, 2010, p. 1180; Wæver, 1995, p. 65).

Huysmans (1998, 2006, 2011), who likewise draws attention to securitization's production of binary categories and antagonistic relations, suggests this is a result of the "politics of fear" in securitization. I share Huysmans' concerns about the identities and relations produced by securitization, and in some respects we are simply using different concepts – fear and threat – to reach the same conclusions. I foreground threat rather than fear, though, because fear is not always present where there is threat: threat can provoke anger, for instance, or bravery (the suppression of fear). But threat (or perception of threat) must be present in order to produce fear. Most importantly, whereas fear draws attention to the emotional state of the securitizing actor or the referent objects of securitization, an analytical focus on threat draws attention to what qualities are ascribed, and how, to that which is excluded from security by virtue of being identified as a threatening Other. In sum, it is threat, specifically, that does the discursive work in securitization, producing both the conditions of possibility for, and limitations within, threat construction and response. To understand how a given securitization becomes possible, we must therefore understand how some issues, objects and populations become thinkable as threats.

The CS acknowledges that the assumed features of an ostensible threat are one of the facilitating conditions of securitization (Buzan, Wæver, & de Wilde, 1998, pp. 32–33), stating that "[i]t is more likely that one can conjure a security threat if certain objects can be referred to that are *generally held to be threatening* – be they tanks, hostile sentiments, or polluted waters" (Buzan et al., 1998, p. 33, emphasis mine), and that "[i]n practice, security is not totally subjective. There are *socially defined limits* to what can and cannot be securitized, although those limits can be changed" (Buzan et al., 1998, p. 39, emphasis mine). This recognition of the durable nature of social meaning and relations (Buzan et al., 1998, pp. 204–206) is often overlooked in accounts that emphasize the CS stance on the radically constructed nature of security without considering its cautions about socially-defined limits, and the implication these have for understanding how securitizations originate, and the practical, empirical limits to security-in-use.

In stating that securitizations are most likely to succeed when they involve things already "generally held to be threatening", the CS suggests that securitizing speech already relies on some degree of prior, intersubjective agreement among securitizing actors and audiences about what objects, populations or states may hold threatening properties, and might plausibly constitute an existential threat. If it is easier to securitize things already "generally held to be threatening", and if there are already, prior to the speech act, "socially defined limits" to what can be securitized, this implies that securitization relies on prior foundational ideas about threat, and these, not the speech act itself, do the ontological work of securitization. That is, securitizing speech is successful when and because there is *already* some consensus that something is (or at least holds latent potential to be) threatening. Therefore, to understand the conditions of possibility in and through which securitizing speech emerges, we need to understand how things come to be "generally held to be threatening" in the first place, who "generally holds" these beliefs, and how this produces the "socially defined limits" of the speech act.

The CS does not take this next analytical step, but its sociological interlocutors suggest that these discursive origins and limits can be found in the historical (Balzacq, 2011; McDonald, 2008) and organizational (Salter, 2008) context of securitization. McDonald (2008) seeks an analytical scope 'beyond the speech act' and 'beyond "the moment"' to determine the conditions within which securitizations become possible, while Balzacq (2011, pp. 3, 14) contends that "every securitization is a historical process" entailing contextual mobilization of "heuristic artefacts (metaphors, policy tools, image repertoires, analogies, stereotypes, emotions, etc.)" that comprise a "semantic repertoire" of security. In addition to the broad historical context of interest to Balzacq and McDonald, Salter (2008) further argues that security has different meanings for actors in different bureaucratic locations, as every organizational context produces its own 'rules of the game' to which securitizing actors must conform in order for their securitizing claims to be heard – that is, to be intelligible and plausible to their audience.

Taken together, these analyses suggest that antecedent threat construction emerges out of historical processes, and works over time to create the discursive conditions and "heuristic artefacts" through and within which things come to be "generally held" to be threatening, and hence ideas about specific security threats become thinkable. Organizational context also produces institutionalized security definitions and practices. Consequently, securitizing actors and their audiences hold prior beliefs about what security and threat 'really mean' in their organization, which then shape how (and where, and to whom) actors can speak security in a manner that is intelligible to their audiences and can support a successful securitizing move. These historical and organizational dynamics work together to produce "socially defined limits" to securitization. This is not an argument against the constructed nature of security threats, but rather that threat construction is initiated, discursively and through bureaucratic structures and practices, long prior to anything identifiable as a securitizing speech act; it is this process and context that makes a given securitization possible. The implication for empirical analysis is that we must attend to contemporary, specific organizational sites within which a given securitization occurs, *and* to longer historical processes of threat construction that necessarily exceed a single place and time.

The argument, then, is that HIV could be securitized, with specific reference to Africa, because both were already "generally held to be threatening" prior to the UNSC sessions. Therefore, to understand how 'HIV is a security threat' became thinkable, and with specific reference to Africa, we must consider the prior claim that HIV is threatening, and discover what foundational assumptions were at work before the UNSC debate in ideas about the nature of the threat posed by HIV, especially in Africa. In other words, we must consider the historical context within which "generally held" ideas about HIV, Africa, threat and security became possible, and the organizational context in which "socially defined limits" to security had already been established by defining security as national or human security and designating it as the responsibility of specific actors in specific organizational locations.

Discursive history: Africa, HIV and threat construction

To trace the discursive conditions in which 'HIV is a security threat' became thinkable, and to identify some inherent constraints of those conditions, we need to consider discourses about HIV, discourses about Africa, and the points at which the two intersect. By tracing the production of "generally held" beliefs about the status of HIV and Africa as threats, and identifying who has held these beliefs, we can discover conceptual overlap and discursive continuity between 'threat' in discourses about HIV, Africa, and security. It is in this conceptual overlap that the idea that HIV is a security threat became 'thinkable' in both national and human security paradigms.

Threat in the discursive history of HIV

Two distinct categories of discourse about HIV have been broadly evident over the course of the pandemic. First is discourse in which PHAs and vulnerable populations are the referent objects, and the needs of these populations are articulated. These have mainly been advanced by social movement activists making broad-based rights and social justice claims. Concepts of threat are generally not evident in these discourses. Second is discourse in which HIV-negative people and lower-prevalence states are the referent objects. These discourses, mainly articulated by those reacting to but not living with HIV, have more frequently invoked notions of 'threat', often locating this threat in high-prevalence states and populations and in HIV-positive people.

HIV has been discursively positioned as exceptional from the earliest years of the pandemic (de Waal, 2006; Ingram, 2013). Crucially, in civil society and activist movements, this discourse and emancipatory praxis has typically conveyed a sense of exceptionalism and urgency *without* explicit invocation of security and threat; calls for action have generally relied on neither the language of security, nor the logic of securitization. Instead, civil society and activist organizations have typically approached treatment access as a human rights and social justice issue (Kapstein & Busby, 2013; Smith & Siplon, 2006), caused by structural violence (Farmer, 2001, 2003) and the inequities of the global political economy (Comaroff, 2007), and requiring structural reform including changes to drugs patents (Kapstein & Busby, 2013; Mugyenyi, 2008) and debt forgiveness (Rustomjee, 2004). Especially when discussing the drivers of the African HIV pandemic, the focus in these analyses is the inter-relationship between African states' marginal status in the global political economy, poverty, gender inequities, and HIV prevalence (Cheru, 2002; de Waal, 2006; Human Rights Watch, 2002; Poku, 2002). Human security claims are in principle possible in these discourses (see for example O'Manique, 2005), but for the most part they have remained latent, displaced by critical social justice analyses that make positive claims reliant not on the invocation of threat, but on what Jean Comaroff (2007, p. 205) calls "repertoires of popular insurgency", entailing a transformative and often radical "health activism".

de Waal (2006, p. 47) for example, describing the work of Ugandan activists, notes their analytical focus on institutionalized discrimination: "They are enraged by specific manifestations of stigma, denial and discrimination in the treatment of people living with HIV and AIDS.... They are also angry about a world order that gives so little value to African lives." In South Africa, the highly successful Treatment Action Campaign (TAC) draws on the tactics and social justice analyses of the anti-apartheid movement, and its demands use the language and logic of human rights and structural reform, not the language of security or the logic of securitization. Typical statements include that "the unnecessary suffering and AIDS related deaths of thousands of people in Africa, Asia and South America [are] human rights violations [and] are the result of poverty and the unaffordability of HIV/AIDS treatment" (Treatment Action Campaign, 2010, p. 6). Supporting this reading of TAC and other community-based activism as not primarily driven by security language or logic, Stephen Lewis (2011) asserts:

> I was five and a half years tramping around Africa [as the UN Special Envoy on AIDS]; I never once heard the word security mentioned, I don't believe it [HIV] was ever considered as a security threat ... I've never seen it as a security threat, I've never met anyone in any of the countries involved, from presidents to activists living with the virus on the ground, who ever cast it in the context of security.

High-prevalence sub-Saharan African states likewise avoided, for the most part, invoking threat in their early responses to HIV. Indeed, with the exception of a small number of states, including Uganda under Museveni and Zambia under Kaunda (Sabatier, 1988), early African state responses to the pandemic were, like state responses elsewhere, rather more underwhelming than urgent (de Waal, 2006, p. 43). But even where African leaders have expressed a sense of urgency, their discourses have not always employed ideas of threat. Kaunda and Mandela, for example, have both spoken about the deaths of their sons due to AIDS (BBC News, 2005; Kaunda, 2004), comparing the fight against HIV and related stigma to the fight against apartheid and colonialism (Kaunda, 2004) and describing lack of treatment access as "a global injustice ... a travesty of human rights on a global scale" (Agence France Presse, 2003).

That these leaders have generally chosen to avoid the language of security may seem counter-intuitive: HIV's material impact on sub-Saharan states would seem to make it eminently 'thinkable' as both a national and human security threat. Yet several authors suggest compelling reasons for African leaders' reticence to employ threat and security discourses when discussing HIV, ranging from resource constraints to racialized boundary institutions to normative concerns about reinforcing images of Africa as dangerous and diseased (de Waal, 2006; Iliffe, 2006; Lieberman, 2009; Nattrass, 2007; Prins, 2004; Sabatier, 1988). Certainly, some African governments did discuss HIV using military metaphors (de Waal, 2006, pp. 106–108), but even these were focused less on elaborating the threat HIV posed to national security, than on using nationalist sentiments to inspire collective social mobilization and to assert state competence and authority (de Waal, 2006, p. 108).

Indeed, the extent to which activist discourses in the late 1990s and 2000s were not couched in the language and logic of security is illustrated in Stephen Lewis' striking statement:

> The driving force in 2000, 2001, 2002, 2003, was treatment. That was the issue. Security had nothing to do with it. People were dying in huge numbers, and the activists were demanding treatment and the people living with AIDS were saying, "We want to stay alive". It was becoming overwhelming ... *questions of security didn't even enter into it, it was just a matter of life and death.*
>
> (Lewis, 2011, emphasis mine)

In his vigorous denunciation of the idea that HIV is a security threat, and his absolute conceptual and rhetorical separation of security from "matters of life and death", Lewis powerfully suggests that actors addressing "a matter of life and death" did not consider themselves to be making security claims or to be operating within security logics or paradigms – even the ostensibly capacious paradigms of human security or security-as-emancipation. He reiterated that during his time (2001–2006) as UN Special Envoy for HIV/AIDS in Africa, "I've never met anyone in any of the countries involved, from presidents to activists living with the virus on the ground, who ever cast it in the context of security", further emphasizing that the people, states and communities most affected by HIV did not express their circumstances or demands in security terms.[1]

Lewis' insistence that treatment access advocacy had "nothing to do" with security reflects that empirically, threat and security, while certainly evident in discourses about HIV in the 1980s and 1990s, were being invoked in ways that were at best in tension with activist claims. In this second category of discourse, which expressed ideas "generally held" by HIV-negative people and lower-prevalence states, it was people living with HIV and higher prevalence states that were constructed as threats. By the mid-1990s, national security observers in the United States had begun to hypothesize that HIV might compromise the political and economic stability of high-prevalence states (Ingram, 2011; McInnes & Rushton, 2010).[2] A 1995 State Department document contended that "[t]he number of AIDS cases will rise rapidly during the remainder of the 1990s and will increasingly undermine other projects intended to foster key US policy goals, including democratization, economic development, conflict resolution and peacekeeping" (U.S. Department of State, 1995, pp. 34–35). Southern African states, where in some cases up to a quarter of the adult population was HIV-positive (Joint United Nations Programme on HIV/AIDS (UNAIDS), 2008), were a central focus of these hypotheses. According to this logic, AIDS mortality would cause population decline, leaving too small a labouring class to support agricultural and industrial production, and too few political and business elites to manage this work. This in turn would lead to sub-optimally functioning economies and political systems, ultimately causing social breakdown, the decline of democratic governance and increased criminality, conflict and power vacuums (Kaplan, 1994; Price-Smith, 1999; U.S. Department of State, 1995). The resulting geopolitical instability would threaten American interests in those regions, thereby constituting a threat to American national security (Fidler, 2003; National Intelligence Council, 2000; U.S. Department of State, 1995; United States Agency for International Development (USAID), 1998).

In discourses where HIV was positioned as a threat to HIV-negative people and lower-prevalence states, it was additionally linked to the putative threat posed by the populations most affected by it, and the behaviours through which the virus is spread. Consider, for example, the contention that HIV

> lies undetected in a person's body for seven, eight, nine, ten years. And since testing is not sufficiently widespread ... 95% of the people in the world who are HIV-positive do not know their status. They are spreading it unintentionally. And therefore, it is the most dangerous disease we've ever seen.
>
> (Holbrooke in Garrett, Piot, & Holbrooke, 2005)

In this construction, HIV is threatening because it cannot be seen, has a long latency period, and thus can be anywhere. But what does it mean for HIV to be anywhere? Unlike air, water or vector-borne diseases, HIV is not simply 'out there' in the environment; it exists only in the human body. Anxiety about the spread of HIV then also betrays anxiety about HIV+ people, constructed as a sinister population of seemingly-healthy people infected with a deadly disease, and spreading it to unsuspecting sero-negative partners. It is a classic articulation of what Sontag (1990, pp. 153–154, 161) calls "[t]he fear of polluting people that AIDS anxiety inevitably communicates...the virus invades the body; the disease... is described as invading the whole society".

In these discourses, the nature of HIV's putative social invasion varies depending upon the population it is linked to. In countries with population-specific epidemics, throughout the 1980s and 1990s HIV was normatively linked to, and epidemiologically prevalent in, populations including gay, bisexual and MSM (men who have sex with men), sex workers, injecting drug users and others with ostensibly deviant sexual and drug use practices – populations constructed as threatening to communities, 'the' family, and religious and cultural values (Sontag, 1990), whose behaviour was coded as uncivilized and unruly, contrary to the orderly, controlled, (re)productive social and economic behaviour that the state requires from citizen-subjects. Even in states with generalized epidemics, HIV was discursively linked to 'outsiders' including minority ethnicities (Lieberman, 2009), but especially sex workers (Booth, 2004) and mobile/migrant populations such as soldiers and long-distance lorry drivers (Iliffe, 2006, pp. 80–81; Sabatier, 1988, p. 115; Treichler, 1999, p. 115). Sexual contact between sex workers, presumed to be female, and mobile populations including soldiers and labourers, presumed to be male, was a particular focus of these discourses, which produced sex workers and migrant populations as 'high risk' subjects. Both groups were considered threatening mainly because they were regarded as vectors through which the virus could move from 'high risk' groups to the 'general population'.

These threat-based discourses work to create binary us/Other, threatened/threatening categories, in which a predominantly HIV-positive population of 'high risk' and morally culpable subjects threatens the health, well-being and security of HIV-negative people. These discourses also work to produce two categories of people living with HIV: morally culpable vectors on one side, and on the other 'innocent victims' not designated as morally responsible for their HIV status, including infants born with HIV (Patton, 1990), recipients of blood transfusions (Shilts, 1988), and faithful wives of "'irresponsible African men' who 'go around' ... and callously bring home infection after infection to their wives" (Booth, 2004, p. 3). Notably, those designated as 'innocent victims' are placed outside of threat constructions and discourses; instead, they are presented as objects of pity, sympathy and charity. The consequence is that some HIV-affected populations are readily thinkable as threats, but that others, including 'faithful wives' and infants, are placed entirely outside the scope of threat-based discourse. Because securitization relies on the invocation of threat, some HIV-affected populations – including female sex workers and migrant men – therefore become much easier to securitize, as they are already "generally held" to be threatening.

Threat in the discursive history of Africa

One can already see that discourses about the threatening nature of HIV over-lapped with and re-inscribed enduring North Atlantic constructions of Africa and Africans as a source of threat. In particular, prior discourses constructing African states and sexuality as Other worked together to produce HIV in Africa as threatening – and did so in a manner that constructed the assumed threat as African, and the threatened referent object as non-African states and peoples.

Multiple theorists have traced the discursive production of Africa as a monolithic Other, constructed in opposition to a North Atlantic self (Fanon, 1967; Mbembe, 2001; Mudimbe, 1988). Africa, in these discourses, is never just a materially existing geographic space; it is also a powerful signifier in the social and political imaginary of the North. This imagined Africa emerges as a signifier and source of disorder, disease and violence, and a place where security, good governance and the Weberian state are largely absent. Discursive construction of African states and governance systems has an extensive history, dating to colonial rule when the prospect of African state independence threatened colonizing states not just for military and economic reasons, but also because this would disrupt racialized hierarchies of states and peoples, and the difference between Africa and Europe that racial rule constructed (Mamdani, 1996). In the 1990s, as American and European strategic interest in Africa receded with the end of the Cold War, discussion of perceived threats emanating from Africa focused on weak, failed and warring states where economic or military intervention might be needed to promote the twin projects of democracy and development, both assumed to be necessary to prevent the effects of poor governance from spilling beyond African borders (Joseph, 1999; Ottaway, 1997).

Mbembe (2006, p. 147) argues that central to these racialized discourses about Africa is

> a discourse on the gap and the lack. It rests on a method of reading the social that consists in simply turning to statistical indices to measure the gap between what the continent is and what we are told it should be.... [T]his method has ended up constructing an image of Africa as a figure of lack.... This is the kind of reading ... that underpins structural adjustment programs, ideologies of good governance and various projects of social engineering.

In this manner, quantitative measurements of HIV prevalence and political stability are deployed to demonstrate that African states lack the capacity, on multiple axes, to respond to the HIV pandemic. Africa is defined by what it is not, and what it is failing to do – and rather than being externally located, the source of this failure is located within the African state. These discourses posit a threatening absence, signified by a lack of good governance, democratic multi-party elections, economic and social development. In turn, high rates of HIV are regarded as both a proximate cause of these weak or absent state attributes, and an ultimate consequence of their absence.[3] Especially, the spread of HIV is thought to be facilitated by 'weak' or 'failed' states (United Nations Economic Commission for Africa, 2008) that lack the power to regulate the behaviours through which HIV is spread.

North Atlantic discourses about 'African sexuality' are another site where Africans have, since the earliest European–African imperial encounters, been constructed as different and therefore threatening (Levine, 2001; Mbembe, 2001, 2006; McClintock, 1995; Packard & Epstein, 1991; Stoler & Cooper, 1997). Gendered, racialized and heteronormative discourses about threatening 'African sexuality' re-emerged in the North in the 1980s and 1990s in two contradictory ways. The first focused on African women's allegedly unregulated fertility, expressing concern that high birth rates and unchecked population growth would cause environmental collapse (Kaplan, 1994; Mathews, 1989). The second expressed fears that uniquely African sexual practices were facilitating the spread of HIV (Caldwell, Caldwell, & Quiggin, 1989). Here, African sexual difference was assumed to be responsible for unleashing the African HIV pandemic, which would lead to AIDS-related deaths and consequent population decline that, it was predicted, would ultimately result in political, economic and social collapse (Kaplan, 1994; Price-Smith, 1999). That these logically incompatible discourses – threat of imminent population explosion and imminent population decline – could exist simultaneously (and that some, like Kaplan's widely-cited "The Coming Anarchy", could espouse both in a single article) indicates the remarkable persistence of the idea that African sexuality itself is inherently threatening to social, economic and political order, and will inevitably produce a problematic number of Africans.

The discursive convergence of HIV, Africa and threat

The construct of 'African AIDS' (Patton, 1990) served to knit together these discourses in which both HIV and Africa had already, through much longer discursive trajectories, been constructed as threatening. To explain why most HIV transmission in sub-Saharan Africa seemed to occur via heterosexual intercourse, and why all of the highest-prevalence states are located in southern Africa, some observers sought a culturally-driven difference in African sexual behaviour (Stillwaggon, 2003). The crudest of these devolved into overtly racist speculation (Nattrass, 2007). Other explanations relating to polygyny, 'widow inheritance' and dry sex (Caldwell et al., 1989; Civic & Wilson, 1996; Kun, 1997; Sow, 1998) did not intentionally reproduce racist tropes, but still drew on stereotypes, assumptions, and impressions of Africa as exotic, exceptional and Other (Stillwaggon, 2003). This re-embedded biomedical and anthropological analyses in long-standing discourses about the threatening nature of Africa – discourses exacerbated by the simultaneous circulation in the 1990s of images from African wars, including Liberian child soldiers, the body of a dead US soldier being dragged through the streets of Mogadishu, and the Rwandan genocide, all of which had the effect of depicting the entire continent as violent and unstable (Hawk, 1992; Karnik, 1998) as well as sexually deviant and diseased (Comaroff, 2007).

Crucially, 'threat' serves as the conceptual lynchpin that unites HIV and Africa across persistent discourses in which Africa is constructed as dangerous, violent and diseased, and equally persistent discourses about HIV in which putatively deviant populations and behaviour are blamed for HIV transmission. In all cases, a desirable ideal (good health, good governance, good citizenship, security) is defined by its absence, and positioned as something threatened by disorder, unregulated appetites, and states too weak or dysfunctional to contain these threats. In the discursive overlap between Africa and threat, the absence of particular state forms and political and economic structures in Africa is interpreted as a security threat to non-African states. In the discursive overlap between HIV and Africa, African sexuality is the common point, and again it is positioned as materially and normatively threatening to non-Africans. 'Threat' enables conceptual linkages between discourses about HIV and Africa, producing a new discursive space wherein the idea 'HIV is a security threat' becomes thinkable, and thinkable with specific reference to other forms of threat (war, disorder, state collapse, unregulated sexuality) already associated with Africa.

The widespread and long-standing circulation of discourses about HIV, Africa and threat does not itself demonstrate that these discourses 'caused' the UNSC debates. But as Malinda Smith (2005, p. 164) argues, "[w]hat is presented as African reality is based on 'truths' that are produced within the discourses themselves.... [T]hese representations help form the policy frames through which the west connects with Africa." Discourses about Africa as a threat, and about HIV as an especially African problem, contributed to "generally held" impressions in the North of Africa and HIV as threatening entities. The aim here is not to draw a causal arrow from these discourses to the UNSC sessions, but to illuminate the widely circulating collection of images, tropes, stereotypes and impressions (Balzacq's (2011) "heuristic artefacts") that formed the broad, historical discursive context of the UNSC sessions, and in particular, to foreground the role that threat plays in these discourses.

The aim is also to illuminate the extent to which human rights, social justice and other emancipatory claims made by civil society activists have tended *not* to employ the language of threat or security. Rather, they have made positive claims that are difficult to articulate in terms of threat. While there is latent possibility for some of these claims to be made in human security terms, social justice and structural violence analyses are not primarily animated by the concept of 'threat'; nor do they tend to employ simple us/Other threatened/threatening binaries. Economic and political systems, structures and power relations are certainly identified as problems to be addressed, but these are not usually constructed as 'threats' existing outside of and in antagonistic, binary opposite relation to a threatened referent object. They are more difficult to express in threat-based logics, including the logics of (liberal) human security and securitization.

Organizational context: the meaning of security in the UN system

Historically produced discourses in which Africa and HIV were already constructed as threatening formed the macro-level discursive terrain in which HIV
became thinkable, with specific reference to Africa, as a security threat; but these
claims were also articulated in an organizational setting in which 'security'
already had an established meaning for securitizing actors. The UN's organizational structure establishes the bounds of what is intersubjectively thinkable and
speakable as a security threat – that is, what securitizing actors and audiences
will mutually accept as intelligible security claims – and provides the organizational, legal and discursive context within which security claims can be made.
This produces a set of enduring constraints that shapes securitizing speech acts,
first by constraining how security threats can be thought and spoken, and second
by constraining where and by whom these claims can be made.

The UN system's policies and organizational structures are premised on
national and to a lesser degree human security. Traditionally, 'security' in the
UN was largely understood to mean national security, that is, the prevention of
war through the maintenance of the territorial integrity of sovereign states. This
is evident in the UN's foundational document, the Charter of the United Nations,
which sets out the normative and functional parameters of the organization, and
which defines the primary purpose of the UN as the prevention of "acts of
aggression or other breaches of the peace" (United Nations, 1945, Article 1.1).
This approach to security dominated in the UN, and especially the UNSC, from
its inception to the end of the Cold War. During this period, the only thinkable
threats to peace and security in the UNSC were military in nature, as empirically
evidenced by the almost exclusive focus of pre-1990 UNSC resolutions on
armed conflict.[4]

As the Cold War came to an end, human security gained increased organizational traction in the UN, appearing in some key policy documents (Boutros-
Ghali, 1992; Commission on Global Governance, 1995; United Nations
Development Programme (UNDP), 1994) as a response to global health,
environmental and other concerns that seemed finally to warrant greater attention. As new conflicts emerged, it was also proffered as the basis of a moral
imperative to protect civilians in conflicts where belligerents had not authorized
UN assistance in brokering a peace. The partial organizational acceptance of
human security discourse in the mid-1990s created opportunities for new securitizing speech acts in the UNSC by expanding the range of 'thinkable' threats
beyond military threats to state security. Empirically, this was evident in the
UNSC's increased rhetorical and sometimes material commitment to matters
somewhat removed from the immediate prevention of armed conflict, and its
authorization of missions and coalition interventions on humanitarian grounds
(Malone, 2004). Still, national security concerns were not simply replaced or
superseded by human security concerns at the end of the Cold War; while the
available discursive space expanded, the functional and normative parameters of

the UNSC's authority continued to be defined by the UN Charter. Securitizing claims made in and by the UNSC still needed to conform to the logic (and legal boundaries) of the Charter, which were defined mainly in national security terms.

The dominance of these definitions of security constitutes a strong "socially defined limit" to what can be securitized, how, in the UN system. Both national and human security approaches make *a priori* assumptions about what constitutes an objectively real threat, to whom, which effectively places securitizing actors in a setting where (1) they must speak and behave as though 'security' has an objective meaning, and (2) the only things that can be securitized are those already "generally held to be threatening" within the logic of national or human security. Consequently, the range of security threats is bounded: within each approach, theoretical and logical parameters render some things simply 'unthinkable' as threats.

In national security approaches, one cannot conceive of disease as a security threat unless a specific disease can be shown to threaten the material and military capabilities, and thus the sovereign existence, of states (Peterson, 2002). This effectively places some diseases and health conditions irrevocably beyond the bounds of security considerations, and ensures that health and illness, writ large, remain discursively, analytically and practically separated from security. It also restricts how and to whom a disease can be understood as threatening, by limiting the referent objects to states and state stability.

Conversely, human security holds the theoretical space to consider threats to individuals and collectivities, and so it can in principle treat a wider range of illnesses as security threats. However, human security still defines security by what is precarious, missing, or threatened. The most common definition of human security is "safety from such chronic threats as hunger, disease, and repression ... [a]nd ... protection from sudden and hurtful disruptions in the pattern of daily life" (United Nations Development Programme (UNDP), 1994). Here, human security is articulated through elaboration of chronic and acute *threats* – not a description of positive entitlements, but a list of things that threaten, hurt and disrupt security. Hence, one must still understand security through reference to threat. This is a subtle boundary condition, but it nevertheless places limits on what can be identified as a human security threat. First, some diseases are more likely to be "generally held" to be threats, and therefore treated as security concerns. This is empirically borne out by the fact that almost all literature linking disease and security focuses on infectious, not chronic disease – even when elaborating what might be read as human security concerns (Brower & Chalk, 2003; Davies, 2008; Garrett, 1996; Peterson, 2002; Price-Smith, 1999; Prins, 2004) – and this is similarly reflected in the 'health security' practices of states, which overwhelmingly focus on infectious rather than chronic disease (Davies, 2010; Feldbaum & Lee, 2004). Second, by requiring the invocation of threat, human security still requires the establishment of binary categories of threatened and threatening subjects, which means actors must still draw on discourses in which some things and people are already "generally held" to be threatening; and their policy responses must still follow the logic of threat containment or eradication. Human security discourse, then, can still enable the exercise of biopolitical and sovereign power (de Larrinaga & Doucet, 2008), as well as the logic of exceptional threat response characteristic of securitization.

In addition to shaping how security can be intelligibly spoken, the organizational structure of the UN system additionally limits where and by whom security claims can be made. The UN body designated as responsible for the maintenance of peace and security, and holding the authority to act in response to international security threats, is the UNSC. It operates as the institutional locus for security matters, that is, the location within which security claims, to be recognized as such by both the organization itself and by its member states, must be made. It also operates as a securitizing actor with the power to articulate securitizing speech acts in the form of UNSC resolutions. Securitizing claims with the power to compel action can only be made in and by the UNSC, and these securitizations and resulting threat response must therefore fall within the UNSC's scope of authority. This limits the form and content of security speech; it also limits who can express it. While any state can request permission to address the UNSC, only the five permanent members (P5) and ten non-permanent members can vote, and only the P5 hold veto power, making these five states by far the most powerful securitizing actors in and of the UNSC. This means that security claims must not only be thinkable and speakable in national or human security terms, but also, if a resolution is sought, these claims must be both intelligible and strategically acceptable to the interests of the P5.

In sum, the conditions of possibility that made HIV thinkable as a security threat also limited the ways in which this threat construction could be expressed. First, both Africa and HIV had already been constructed as threatening through widely circulating, historically produced global North discourses. Second, within the UN system, 'security' was already understood to mean national or human security, and was associated with specific locations, actors, and security practices. The discursive context was one in which Africa, HIV, and HIV in Africa were already "generally held" to be threatening in the North Atlantic imaginary; this, in combination with an organizational context that already limited security concerns to national or human security, created the "socially defined limits" to how HIV as a security threat could be thought and spoken.

Conclusion

This chapter has argued that securitization of a given issue becomes thinkable when conceptual linkages can be made across discourses in which some people, places and issues have already historically been constructed as threatening; and that these 'thinkable' securitizations must then be spoken in a context (usually organizational) in which security already has agreed-upon meaning for actors. Thus 'threat' could conceptually unite discourses about HIV and Africa because both had already, separately, been explicitly discursively positioned as threatening in national security terms, and held latent potential to be positioned as threatened in human security terms.

The discourses that make HIV as a security threat 'thinkable' create both possibilities and constraints. Ideationally and normatively, HIV became 'thinkable' as a national security threat because in discourses about HIV and Africa it was already "generally held" to be threatening, and prevalent in threatening places and populations. These discourses relied on and reinforced racialized, gendered notions about Africa (and especially its sex workers and soldiers) as threatening, and aligned closely with national security concerns about violent conflict, and political, economic and social collapse within and across African states. Yet the discourses of human security also offered alluring latent possibilities. Prior to the UNSC debate, the language of threat and security was not generally invoked in ASO, activist and PHA discourse, but the concerns they expressed did in principle align with those of human security. There remained the latent possibility, then, of using human security claims in an effort to draw increased attention and resources to HIV and thereby transform the global response.

These security discourses would shape two different and not fully compatible sets of ideas about how and why HIV was a security threat and what policy responses ought to be undertaken. This is not, of course, a deterministic process: discourses can be contested, and multiple conflicting discourses about a single entity can exist at the same time. While the idea that HIV was a security threat was made *possible* by the discourses described here, it was not inevitable. As the next chapter will demonstrate, there would continue to be tension between discursive links between HIV, security and Africa; a highly resilient UN organizational structure that continues to privilege a particular vision of security; and the ambition of some global health actors to achieve normative change by framing HIV as a security threat with a view to transforming the global HIV response.

Notes

1 Of course, some activists may have tacitly supported, or at least not opposed, use of security rhetoric and securitization strategies; it is possible that they, like other securitizing actors, hoped securitization would have some strategic utility. But the language, grammar, tactics and political analysis that TAC and other activist groups explicitly expressed and endorsed were overwhelmingly *not* those of security and securitization.

2 These were influenced by historical analyses of instances of political and economic relations, balances of power among states and domestic political structures being altered by infectious disease (Diamond, 1997; McNeill, 1998), and post-Cold War interest in the relationship between infectious disease, politics and economics in a highly networked and interdependent world (Barnett & Whiteside, 2006; Brower & Chalk, 2003; Chalk, 2006; Peterson, 2002; Price-Smith, 1999; United States Agency for International Development (USAID), 1998).

3 See also Abrahamsen's (2005) argument that Africa has been securitized as a threat post-9/11, especially with reference to weak/failed states thought to provide haven for terrorists.

4 The exceptions are resolutions relating to the admission of new UN members as former colonies gained independence, and resolutions concerning apartheid in South Africa,

some of which expressed concern about state repression of protestors and execution of political prisoners. (Both of these are still consistent with national security concern for state sovereignty, in the first case, and regional stability and security, in the second.)

References

Abrahamsen, Rita. (2005). Blair's Africa: The politics of securitization and fear. *Alternatives, 30*(1), 55–80.

Agence France Presse. (2003). Mandela steals show at Paris AIDS meeting. Retrieved 20 October 2013 from www.commondreams.org/headlines03/0714-07.htm.

Aradau, Claudia. (2004). Security and the democratic scene: desecuritization and emancipation. *Journal of International Relations and Development, 7*(4), 388–413.

Balzacq, Thierry. (2011). A theory of securitization: origins, core assumptions, variants. In Thierry Balzacq (Ed.), *Securitization Theory: How Security Problems Emerge and Dissolve* (pp. 1–30). New York: Routledge.

Barnett, Tony & Whiteside, Alan. (2006). *AIDS in the Twenty-First Century: Disease and Globalization* (2nd edn). New York: Palgrave Macmillan.

BBC News. (2005). Mandela's eldest son dies of Aids. Retrieved 20 October 2013 from http://news.bbc.co.uk/2/hi/africa/4151159.stm.

Booth, Karen M. (2004). *Local Women, Global Science: Fighting AIDS in Kenya*. Bloomington, IN: Indiana University Press.

Boutros-Ghali, Boutros. (1992). *An Agenda for Peace*. New York: United Nations.

Brower, Jennifer & Chalk, Peter. (2003). *The Global Threat of New and Reemerging Infectious Diseases: Reconciling US National Security and Public Health Policy*. Virginia: RAND.

Buzan, Barry, Wæver, Ole, & de Wilde, Jaap. (1998). *Security: A New Framework for Analysis*. Boulder, CO: Lynne Rienner.

Caldwell, John C., Caldwell, Pat, & Quiggin, Pat. (1989). The social context of AIDS in sub-Saharan Africa. *Population and Development Review, 15*(2), 185–234.

Chalk, Peter. (2006). Disease and the complex processes of securitization in the Asia-Pacific. In Mely Caballero-Anthony, Ralf Emmers & Amitav Acharya (Eds.), *Non-Traditional Security in Asia: Dilemmas in Securitization* (pp. 112–135). Aldershot: Ashgate.

Charter of the United Nations and Statute of the International Court of Justice, United Nations Department of Public Information (1945 [26 June 1945]).

Cheru, Fantu. (2002). Debt, adjustment and the politics of effective response to HIV/AIDS in Africa. *Third World Quarterly, 23*(2), 299–312.

Civic, Diane & Wilson, David. (1996). Dry sex in Zimbabwe and implications for condom use. *Social Science & Medicine, 42*(1), 91–98.

Comaroff, Jean. (2007). Beyond bare life: AIDS (bio)politics and the neoliberal order. *Public Culture, 19*(1), 197–219.

Commission on Global Governance. (1995). *Our Global Neighbourhood: The Report of the Commission on Global Governance*. Oxford: Oxford University Press.

Davies, Sara E. (2008). Securitizing infectious disease. *International Affairs, 84*(2), 295–313.

Davies, Sara E. (2010). What contribution can International Relations make to the evolving global health agenda? *International Affairs, 86*(5), 1167–1190.

de Larrinaga, Miguel & Doucet, Marc G. (2008). Sovereign power and the biopolitics of human security. *Security Dialogue, 39*(5), 517–537.

de Waal, Alexander. (2006). *AIDS and Power: Why There Is No Political Crisis – Yet.* New York: Zed Books.

Diamond, Jared. (1997). *Guns, Germs and Steel: The Fates of Human Societies.* New York: W.W. Norton & Co.

Fanon, Frantz. (1967). *Black Skin, White Masks* (Charles Lam Markmann, Trans.). New York: Grove Press.

Farmer, Paul. (2001). *Infections and Inequalities: The Modern Plagues.* Berkeley, CA: University of California Press.

Farmer, Paul. (2003). *Pathologies of Power: Health, Human Rights and the New War on the Poor.* Berkeley, CA: University of California Press.

Feldbaum, Harley & Lee, Kelley. (2004). Public health and security. In Alan Ingram (Ed.), *Health, Foreign Policy and Security: Towards a Conceptual Framework for Research and Policy (UK Global Health Programme Working Paper #2)* (pp. 19–28). London: Nuffield Trust & UK Global Health Programme.

Fidler, David P. (2003). Racism or *realpolitik*? US foreign policy and the HIV/AIDS catastrophe in sub-Saharan Africa. *Journal of Gender Race & Justice, 7*(1), 97–146.

Foucault, Michel. (2002 [1970]). *The Order of Things* (Tavistock/Routledge, Trans.). Abingdon: Routledge.

Garrett, Laurie. (1996). The return of infectious diseases. *Foreign Affairs, 75*(1), 66–79.

Garrett, Laurie, Piot, Peter, & Holbrooke, Richard C. (2005). *HIV and National Security.* Paper presented at the panel discussion organized by the Council on Foreign Relations.

Hawk, Beverly G. (1992). Introduction: metaphors of African coverage. In Beverly G. Hawk (Ed.), *Africa's Media Image* (pp. 3–14). New York: Praeger.

Human Rights Watch. (2002). Suffering in silence: the links between human rights abuses and HIV transmission to girls in Zambia. New York: Human Rights Watch.

Huysmans, Jef. (1998). Security! What do you mean? From concept to thick signifier. *European Journal of International Relations, 4*(2), 226–255.

Huysmans, Jef. (2006). *The Politics of Insecurity: Fear, Migration and Asylum in the EU.* New York: Routledge.

Huysmans, Jef. (2011). What's in an act? On security speech acts and little security nothings. *Security Dialogue, 45*(4–5), 371–383.

Iliffe, John. (2006). *The African AIDS Epidemic: A History.* Oxford: James Currey Ltd.

Ingram, Alan. (2011). The Pentagon's HIV/AIDS programmes: governmentality, political economy, security. *Geopolitics, 16*(3), 655–674.

Ingram, Alan. (2013). After the exception: HIV/AIDS beyond salvation and scarcity. *Antipode, 45*(2), 436–454.

Joint United Nations Programme on HIV/AIDS (UNAIDS). (2008). 2008 report on the global AIDS epidemic. Geneva: Joint United Nations Programme on HIV/AIDS (UNAIDS).

Joseph, Richard (Ed.). (1999). *State, Conflict and Democracy in Africa.* Boulder, CO: Lynne Rienner.

Kaplan, Robert D (1994). The coming anarchy. *The Atlantic Monthly, 273*(2), 44–76.

Kapstein, Ethan B. & Busby, Joshua W. (2013). *AIDS Drugs for All: Social Movements and Market Transformations.* Cambridge, UK: Cambridge University Press.

Karnik, Niranjan S. (1998). Rwanda & the media: imagery, war & refuge. *Review of African Political Economy, 25*(78), 611–623.

Kaunda, Kenneth. (2004). *Opening Remarks by His Excellency Dr. Kenneth D. Kaunda.* Paper presented at the African Development Forum IV: Governance for a Progressing Africa, Addis Ababa.

Kun, K. E. (1997). Female genital mutilation: the potential for increased risk of HIV infection. *International Journal of Gynecology and Obstetrics, 59*(1997), 153–155.

Levine, Philippa. (2001). Public health, venereal disease and colonial medicine in the later nineteenth century. In Roger Davidson & Lesley A. Hall (Eds.), *Sex, Sin and Suffering: Venereal Disease and European Society Since 1870* (pp. 160–172). London: Routledge.

Lewis, Stephen (2011, 17 January). (Personal interview with author.)

Lieberman, Evan. (2009). *Boundaries of Contagion: How Ethnic Politics Have Shaped Government Responses to AIDS.* New Jersey: Princeton University Press.

Malone, David M. (Ed.). (2004). *The UN Security Council: From the Cold War to the 21st Century.* Boulder, CO: Lynne Rienner.

Mamdani, Mahmood. (1996). *Citizen and Subject: Contemporary Africa and the Legacy of Late Colonialism.* Princeton: Princeton University Press.

Mathews, Jessica Tuchman. (1989). Redefining security. *Foreign Affairs, 68*(2), 162–177.

Mbembe, Achille. (2001). *On the Postcolony* (A. M. Berrett, Janet Roitman, Murray Last, & Steven Rendall, Trans.). Berkeley, CA: University of California Press.

Mbembe, Achille. (2006). *On the Postcolony*: a brief response to critics. *African Identities, 4*(2), 143–178.

McClintock, Anne. (1995). *Imperial Leather: Race, Gender and Sexuality in the Colonial Contest.* New York: Routledge.

McDonald, Matt. (2002). Human security and the construction of security. *Global Society, 16*(3), 277–295.

McDonald, Matt. (2008). Securitization and the construction of security. *European Journal of International Relations, 14*(4), 563–587.

McInnes, Colin & Rushton, Simon. (2010). HIV, AIDS and security: where are we now? *International Affairs, 86*(1), 225–245.

McNeill, William H. (1998). *Plagues and Peoples.* New York: Anchor Books.

Mudimbe, V. Y. (1988). *The Invention of Africa: Gnosis, Philosophy and the Order of Knowledge.* Bloomington, IN: Indiana University Press.

Mugyenyi, Peter. (2008). *Genocide By Denial: How Profiteering From HIV/AIDS Killed Millions.* Kampala: Fountain Publishers.

National Intelligence Council. (2000). The global infectious disease threat and its implications for the United States. Langley: National Intelligence Council.

Nattrass, Nicoli. (2007). *Mortal Combat: AIDS Denialism and the Struggle for Antiretrovirals in South Africa.* Scottsville: University of KwaZulu-Natal Press.

O'Manique, Colleen. (2005). The "securitisation" of HIV/AIDS in sub-Saharan Africa: a critical feminist lens. *Policy and Society, 24*(1), 24–47.

Ottaway, Marina (Ed.). (1997). *Democracy in Africa: The Hard Road Ahead.* Boulder, CO: Lynne Rienner.

Packard, Randall M. & Epstein, Paul. (1991). Epidemiologists, social scientists, and the structure of medical research on AIDS in Africa. *Journal of Social Science and Medicine, 33*(7), 771–794.

Patton, Cindy. (1990). *Inventing AIDS.* New York: Routledge.

Peterson, Susan. (2002). Epidemic disease and national security. *Security Studies, 12*(2), 43–81.

Piot, Peter. (2012). *No Time To Lose: A Life In Pursuit of Deadly Viruses.* New York: W.W. Norton.

Poku, Nana K. (2002). Poverty, debt and Africa's HIV/AIDS crisis. *International Affairs, 78*(3), 531–546.

Price-Smith, Andrew T. (1999). Ghosts of Kigali: infectious disease and global stability at the turn of the century. *International Journal*, *54*(3), 426–442.

Prins, Gwyn. (2004). AIDS and global security. *International Affairs*, *80*(5), 931–952.

Rothschild, Emma. (1995). What is security? *Daedalus*, *124*(3), 53–98.

Rustomjee, Cyrus. (2004). Jubilee South Africa: a case study for the UKZN project entitled: Globalisation, marginalisation and new social movements in post-apartheid South Africa. Durban: The Centre for Civil Society and the School of Development Studies, University of KwaZulu-Natal.

Sabatier, Renée. (1988). *Blaming Others: Prejudice, Race and Worldwide AIDS*. Philadelphia, PA: New Society Publishers.

Salter, Mark B. (2008). Securitization and desecuritization: a dramaturgical analysis of the Canadian Air Transport Security Authority. *Journal of International Relations and Development*, *11*(4), 321–349.

Shilts, Randy. (1988). *And the Band Played On: Politics, People and the AIDS Epidemic*. New York: Penguin Books.

Smith, Malinda. (2005). The constitution of Africa as a security threat. *Review of Constitutional Studies*, *10*(1), 163–206.

Smith, Raymond A. & Siplon, Patricia D. (2006). *Drugs Into Bodies: Global AIDS Treatment Activism*. Westport, CT: Praeger.

Sontag, Susan. (1990). *Illness as Metaphor and AIDS and its Metaphors*. New York: Picador.

Sow, P.S. et al. (1998). Pratiques traditionelles et transmission de l'infection à VIH au Sénégal: l'exemple du lévirat et du sororat. *Médecine et Maladies Infectieuses*, *28*(2), 203–205.

Stillwaggon, Eileen. (2003). Racial metaphors: interpreting sex and AIDS in Africa. *Development and Change*, *34*(5), 809–832.

Stoler, Ann Laura & Cooper, Frederick. (1997). Between metropole and colony: rethinking a research agenda. In Ann Laura Stoler & Frederick Cooper (Eds.), *Tensions of Empire: Colonial Cultures in a Bourgeois World* (pp. 1–56). Berkeley, CA: University of California Press.

Treatment Action Campaign. (2010). *Fighting For Our Lives: The History of the Treatment Action Campaign 1998–2010*. Cape Town: Treatment Action Campaign.

Treichler, Paula A. (1999). *How to Have Theory in an Epidemic: Cultural Chronicles of AIDS*. Durham, NC: Duke University Press.

U.S. Department of State. (1995). U.S. International Strategy on HIV/AIDS. Retrieved 8 November 2012 from http://dosfan.lib.uic.edu/ERC/environment/releases/9507.html.

Ullman, Richard. (1983). Redefining security. *International Security*, *8*(1), 129–153.

United Nations Children's Fund (UNICEF), & World Health Organization (WHO). (2009). Diarrhoea: why children are still dying and what can be done: UNICEF and WHO.

United Nations Development Programme (UNDP). (1994). *Human Development Report 1994*. New York: Oxford University Press.

United Nations Economic Commission for Africa. (2008). *Securing Our Future: Report of the Commission on HIV/AIDS and Governance in Africa*. Geneva: Commission on HIV/AIDS and Governance in Africa.

United States Agency for International Development (USAID). (1998). Reducing the threat of infectious diseases of major public health importance: USAID's initiative to prevent and control infectious diseases. Retrieved 6 November 2012 from www.usaid.gov/our_work/global_health/id/idstrategy.pdf.

Wæver, Ole. (1995). Securitization and desecuritization. In Ronnie D. Lipschutz (Ed.), *On Security* (pp. 46–86). New York: Columbia University Press.

4 Speech acts, framing contests and strategic action in HIV securitization[1]

The speech act is the moment of articulation alerting us that a securitization is underway. This articulation is at once the product of underlying assumptions shaped by prior, historically-produced discourses and threat constructions; the deliberate, strategic actions of securitizing actors; and effects of particular organizational contexts. Speech acts then trigger contestation as actors debate the meaning of a given invocation of existential threat, the appropriate referent object, and the proper form of threat response. All of these become partially fixed as actors settle on a course of action, usually expressed in the form of a high-level policy directive, but framing contests are rife with never fully-resolved tensions and possibilities. The entire process, however, operates in and is shaped by both the logic of securitization, and the context within which securitizing speech emerges.

This chapter explores the dynamics of securitizing strategies, speech and framing contests in international HIV securitization, with a view to identifying the presence and effects – the creative potential, tensions and constraints – of securitization logic in the organizational context of the UN. First it assesses the explanations of two key policy leaders, Richard Holbrooke and Peter Piot, of how they were persuaded, and persuaded others, that HIV was (or should be framed as) a security threat and should be discussed by the UNSC. Examining the foundational assumptions underpinning their articulations of the relationship between HIV, Africa and security shows that, from the outset, the idea 'HIV is a security threat' held different meanings and rested, in different forms, on the discourses explored in the previous chapter. Second, the chapter explores strategies, in the form of creative diplomacy and use of evidence, that securitizing actors employed to create the conditions for a successful securitizing speech act in a specific political and organizational context. Third, the chapter analyses this securitizing speech as a framing contest in which competing narratives were articulated, but in which the combined logic of securitization and organizational imperatives of the UN began inexorably to shape the ultimate outcome. This analysis entails close reading of the UNSC discussions to reveal policy problem and solution framing contests reflecting different interpretations of the relationship between HIV, security, Africa and peacekeepers: one rooted in national security, focused on prevention programmes in the security sector, the other rooted in human security, and entailing broader redistributive strategies and investments to support treatment access. The resulting meaning-making contests, while never fully resolved, were nevertheless constrained by the logic of securitization, especially as it took specific form in the UNSC context, and ultimately produced a relatively narrow securitization and threat response. The chapter concludes by summarizing how securitization logic, especially threat construction and response, worked to produce this outcome. To be clear, the argument is not that the UNSC sessions and Resolution 1308 'did nothing'; the point is to understand what *securitization* did and how it worked in this instance.

Converging means and divergent ends in the securitization of HIV

In the UN system, UNAIDS Executive Director Peter Piot and US Ambassador to the UN Richard Holbrooke were among the primary sources and strongest advocates of the idea that HIV was a security problem warranting UNSC attention. Each had a complex set of motivations for positioning HIV as a security threat, and their ethical and instrumental reasoning, as well as their organizational locations, led them to articulate two different understandings of the ways in which HIV constituted a security threat. These would give rise to multiple framing contests when the UNSC eventually discussed HIV.

Piot and Holbrooke were not, alone, responsible for HIV securitization, nor did they single-handedly craft these competing narratives. Rather, both were highly visible leaders whose public statements about HIV, Africa and security represented the positions of two larger constituencies, and who endeavoured to persuade others by appealing to shared understandings. As such, their articulated ideas are a meaningful empirical indicator of underlying, intersubjectively held assumptions that drove HIV securitization in the UNSC. Put differently, their statements and strategies offer a grounded means of exploring how the widely held sentiment that there was an urgent need to 'do something' about HIV – a sentiment that was driving the entire global response and that would soon catalyse bigger political shifts – manifested when expressed in the UN system, refracted through the lens of security and the strategies of securitization.

When he became Executive Director of UNAIDS in 1996, Piot wanted to transform the global response to HIV, in part by moving it from the domain of traditional global public health actors – WHO, health-focused NGOs, and national ministries of health – to what he perceived to be more powerful decision-making tables. His stated ambition was to attract greater funding for HIV and improve treatment access in the developing world (Piot, 2009). He recalls,

> I was wondering, "How long can we document the catastrophe that's unfolding?" ... I said, "I want to change the world, I want to have an impact." I was convinced that we needed to reposition AIDS.... And one of the things that I'd learned in politics is there are only two things that matter at the end of the day, I think, and that's the economy and security, and the

rest ... "c'est la literature", you know. And so I thought we need to reposition it, and get out of the ghetto of AIDS doctors and AIDS activists, usually fighting with each other, and change the conversation. And put it on the top political agenda. If it's not at the top of the political agenda, then there won't be the resources, there won't be the courageous decisions that are needed.

(Piot, 2009)

The decision to bring HIV to the UNSC was "on the simple grounds of, looking at the UN, what is taken seriously, where is the power? It's the Security Council, so we go for the Security Council. I mean, there was absolutely no theory behind it" (Piot, 2009). Principled belief that the global response to HIV required transformation thus led to strategic action to attract attention and resources by positioning the virus as a security problem.[2]

Having determined to frame HIV as a security matter, Piot (2009)

started looking at AIDS as a purely political issue, not as a medical issue. It makes a huge difference, how you approach it. Because in politics I said, OK, where do we want to go, what's our strategy, and what are the alliances to get, who are our friends, who are our enemies?

Piot's senior advisors identified Holbrooke as an important ally. In part this simply reflects that the US is a major UN donor and a permanent member of the UNSC, and would need to be on side with any efforts to discuss HIV in that forum. Pursuit of this alliance was also facilitated because several senior staff in UNAIDS had personal and professional ties to senior staff in the White House and the US Permanent Mission to the UN (Knight, 2008, p. 48), giving them privileged access to political and diplomatic staff, including Holbrooke. There followed a series of meetings between Piot, Holbrooke and their advisors between 1998–2000 (Knight, 2008, p. 105).

Piot recalls that in addition to meetings, UNAIDS employed other strategies to persuade Holbrooke that HIV was a security issue:

PP: Holbrooke made a trip to Central Africa ... to look at security issues. And I had met him before to brief him a bit on AIDS in the countries he was visiting – it was Rwanda, Burundi, the Great Lakes. And *I had also made sure that wherever he would go, there would be a person with HIV, and there would be somebody from UNAIDS* there. So we had organized that. And he came back and he said, "Oh my god, this is a big problem, AIDS."

SH: And did you know at that point that he was scheduled for the next rotation of President of the Security Council?

PP: Yes. Yeah, yeah, you always have to do your homework for who is when, and all that. So he said, and that was his idea ... in January we [the US] have the Presidency, it's going to be Africa we want to highlight, and he said, let's have a debate on AIDS.

(Piot, 2009, emphasis mine)

This indicates a deliberate effort to engage Holbrooke through experiential learning in the form of face-to-face encounters with people living with and affected by HIV. Describing these encounters, which included meeting Namibian women who "had gotten HIV from their husbands" (Sternberg, 2002) and a visit to a day centre for AIDS orphans, Holbrooke (in PBS, 2006) recalled:

> I didn't need the trip to Africa to know AIDS was a huge problem, but you have to see it on the ground firsthand in detail to understand all its dimensions. Watching kids sleep in the gutters in Lusaka ... knowing that they will become either prostitutes or rape victims, either getting or spreading the disease, because there's no shelter for them, and that the government is doing nothing about it, makes a powerful impression on you.

Holbrooke's experience indeed appears to have triggered a strong reaction: he cited it as the catalyst for his decision to put HIV on the UNSC agenda (Sternberg, 2002), since "AIDS is a security issue because it's destroying the security, the stability of countries" (Holbrooke in PBS, 2006). Initial moves to securitize HIV, then, involved not just linguistic but *material* engagement with the world. The strategic use of people living with HIV to persuade and educate Holbrooke, with the ultimate aim of provoking moral action, affirms that securitization is not solely accomplished through speech acts; rather speech acts emerge out of prior discursive and material contexts and encounters.

It also affirms that even these early moves, intended precisely to build a relationship between a securitizing actor and people living with HIV, meant to be understood as threatened, triggered the production of threatening as well as threatened HIV-affected subjects. In interpreting orphaned children as either prostitutes or rape victims, Holbrooke posits categories of vulnerable, threatened victims who "get" HIV, and culpable threatening subjects who "spread" it; of raped people, who are victims, and of prostitutes, who are presumably neither raped nor victims. The binary logic of us/them, threatened/threatening and inside/outside that characterizes securitization, and echoes the gendered, threat-based discourses considered in the previous chapter, was present even in an encounter meant specifically to produce empathy and solidarity.

Furthermore, in spite of Holbrooke's contention that this experience was the catalyst for the UNSC sessions, this narrative does not tell the full story. Holbrooke's perception that HIV was a security threat predated his African trip and involved his interpretation of a different social phenomenon and different social bodies. Specifically, while his visit to southern Africa may have persuaded him that HIV was a problem *in Africa*, he already held the belief that HIV was a problem *in peacekeeping*. Holbrooke had as early as 1992 become convinced that UN peacekeepers were responsible for spreading HIV in countries where they had been deployed. In a 2006 interview, he remarked,

> in Cambodia in 1992 ... I went there as a private citizen, and I saw the peacekeepers from the UN in Cambodia, and they were doing a good job.

But at night I saw them wandering around the street drunk and going into whorehouses and so on and so forth, and I was quite upset about this. It was clear that they were spreading AIDS, and they were going to take AIDS back with them. So I wrote a letter to the head of the UN in Cambodia saying, "You've really got to do something about this", and I never got a reply. But it stuck with me, and then when I became ambassador to the UN seven years later, that was a seminal memory in my mind.

(PBS, 2006)

In more cautious diplomatic language, Holbrooke also shared this experience in the July 2000 UNSC session, saying:

I was disturbed by the fact that the United Nations forces were already spreading AIDS. I was so disturbed, in fact, that on 27 July 1992, as a private citizen, I wrote a letter to [UN representatives].... On that date, I wrote something which, if one changed the name "Cambodia" to the words "certain countries in Africa where peacekeepers are", would be true today.

(Holbrooke in United Nations Security Council, 2000a)

Holbrooke's recounting of his experience in Cambodia in at least two public spaces suggests that over a 14-year period from 1992–2006, he consistently held the belief that peacekeepers and sex workers were "spreading AIDS", undermining HIV prevention and peacebuilding efforts. His Cambodian encounter, while also an instance of experiential learning, involved not a deliberate, curated meeting with people living with HIV, but rather the incidental witnessing of what Holbrooke considered dangerous behaviours and sites of contagion: drunk, sexually promiscuous soldiers, and "whorehouses" and their inhabitants, many of whom were diseased or about to become so. In contrast to the women and orphans introduced to him by UNAIDS, who were constructed as threatened, these peacekeepers and sex workers and their assumed HIV status were understood as *threatening* to state-building and peacekeeping efforts.

Holbrooke's encounters in southern Africa did also produce a response aligned with Piot's and UNAIDS' expectations: he characterized the trip as "heartbreaking" (Sternberg, 2002), and would later, as CEO of the Global Business Coalition on HIV, advocate for corporate investment in the global HIV response. But he clearly had a prior interpretation of the relationship between HIV, peacekeeping, and sex work, particularly that "prostitutes" and peacekeepers were dangerous vectors of HIV transmission. Furthermore, in contending that HIV was a security threat because it threatened "the stability of countries", even his initial response to HIV in Africa was framed in national security terms wherein the unregulated behaviour of soldiers and sex workers was dangerous to the state, which itself became the threatened referent object.

Holbrooke additionally intended for the UNSC debate to advance a separate domestic political agenda. Al Gore, then US Vice-President, had begun his presidential campaign, and his supporters, including Holbrooke, were keen to provide him with opportunities to articulate his foreign policy vision in an international forum (David, 2001, pp. 578–579). Gore's domestic campaign had also been the target of activist "zaps" protesting the US administration's backing of pharmaceutical companies' patents on new antiretroviral treatments (Kapstein & Busby, 2013, pp. 128–129). The timing of Holbrooke's rotation as UNSC president was thus fortuitous for Democratic strategists, as Holbrooke could use his position to invite Gore to speak about HIV, simultaneously placating domestic activists and demonstrating his foreign policy capabilities. Indeed, Gore would use this platform to announce several funding initiatives. These were planned or already-committed funds, all determined well before the UNSC sessions, but announcing the funding publically in the UNSC contributed to perceptions, at home and abroad, that the US and Gore were acting to address HIV.

In sum, Holbrooke, Piot, and the constituencies they represented had ambitious but stalled agendas prior to the UNSC debate. Holbrooke had been unable through unilateral personal action to persuade UN and troop-contributing countries to regulate peacekeepers' sexual conduct, and also wanted to advance Gore's presidential bid. Piot and UNAIDS had been unable to place HIV "at the top of the political agenda" in order to trigger substantial reallocation of resources. Having been unable to achieve these goals in isolation, each found in the other a useful ally. This complicates narratives that suggest Holbrooke was the prime mover of international HIV securitization in the UNSC, and that this was simply an expression of an earlier US-based securitization that was then promoted internationally (McInnes & Rushton, 2013; Sjöstedt, 2011). To be sure, US power had a role to play, as it does in many international political events, but Piot and his advisors had their own agenda, acted to further that agenda independently of the US, and would continue to do so over the course of the next decade.

What is at work here is a jointly coordinated state-IO action to advance the idea that HIV is a security threat, and to place it on the UNSC agenda. This affirms that contrary to realist premises, even in the apparently state-centric world of international security, and even in the UNSC composed exclusively of nation-states, the state cannot be the sole unit of analysis. Professional and personal networks mattered deeply in the construction of HIV as a security threat, and these networks operated across state and IO lines, even at the highest levels of policy-making. Yet, in contrast to a tendency in some social movement literature to gloss IO and civil society actors as motivated by moral or principled beliefs and state actors as motivated by strategic concerns, this case suggests that *both* state and IO representatives were motivated by *both* principled and strategic concerns.

However, while bringing HIV to the UNSC may have been a cooperative action, only some parts of these agendas were convergent. While sharing the idea that there was a relationship between HIV and security, Piot and Holbrooke differed in their articulated understanding of how 'HIV is a security threat' should be interpreted, and in the change they hoped to effect by bringing HIV to the UNSC. As the narrator of *The Autobiography of Alice B. Toklas* says when recounting two friends' versions of their quarrel, "They told exactly the same story only it was different, very different" (Stein, 1960 [1933], p. 123). Even at this stage, there was a broader and narrower agenda: Piot's ambition to transform the global response to HIV and improve treatment access, and Holbrooke's stated objective to regulate the sexual conduct of peacekeepers. Securitization efforts would ultimately prove to be far more effective at advancing the narrower of these agendas.

The drivers of principled and strategic action

These two articulations about why HIV should be understood as a security threat are underpinned by different underlying assumptions. While not always explicitly articulated in the process of constructing HIV as a security threat, these assumptions are nevertheless required for the frames to make sense, and excavating them can help us understand the logic at work in each.

The UNAIDS narrative articulated by Piot began with the position that HIV was a catastrophe needing increased attention and resources, and that to acquire these, the matter needed to be brought to more powerful decision-making tables. For a security response to HIV to make sense in this articulation, we first need to believe that greater attention and resources are needed for HIV – a position well-supported empirically in 2000. Similarly, the devastating impact of HIV has been well-documented, though there was no *a priori* reason to believe that this devastation necessitated the securitization of HIV. The conclusion that *securitization*, specifically, is warranted, rests on assumptions about security, particularly that security is inherently more powerful than health. The two ideas that HIV was a catastrophe and that security matters most resulted in classic Copenhagen-style securitization logic: political systems deal with "politics as usual" and are not equipped to deal with complex catastrophes such as HIV. These require an extraordinary response in excess of the capabilities of health actors, and immediate action rather than prolonged debate between activists, public health actors, and politicians. Security mechanisms are designed precisely to deal with extraordinary crises by taking immediate, decisive action, and have the power, authority and resources to do so. Therefore HIV should be understood as an appropriate matter for security actors, since they have the resources to address large-scale crises and the authority to compel urgent action.

The assessment that rather than reallocating resources and authority from security systems to health systems, the preferable solution at least in the short term is to redefine the scope of health and security actor responsibilities such that HIV becomes a security threat, and thus the responsibility of security actors, has perhaps necessitated longer-term trade-offs. That is, the analysis represents a partial insight into a deeply problematic ordering of international priorities, global health and security work, and socio-economic structures, but ultimately it reinforces precisely that which it began by critiquing: the privileging of security over health. As Ingram (2013) suggests, this risks producing a temporary exceptional response to a single health crisis, while leaving intact the structural drivers and neoliberal logics at the core of global health inequities. Further, as argued in the previous chapter, casting HIV in the national and human security terms dominant in the UN requires threat construction, and thus production of the binaries and hierarchies that characterize securitization.

The assumptions underpinning the peacekeeping narrative articulated by Holbrooke, while also culminating in the contention that HIV is a security threat, are different. Whereas Piot's analysis began with a critique of traditional security and global health practices and political priorities, Holbrooke's statements about peacekeepers began with implicit acceptance of those practices and priorities. The assertion that HIV is a security threat because peacekeepers' behaviour spreads HIV and further destabilizes fragile states, rests on and reinforces traditional national security preoccupations with war, states and sovereign territoriality. Additionally, assertions about how peacekeepers were spreading HIV rest on the assumption that peacekeepers are male, heterosexual, possessing sexual agency, and at risk because of unprotected sexual relations with women, mainly sex workers. In the quote cited above, the presumably female sex workers in Cambodia are all but erased (Holbrooke refers to "whorehouses" but not the women who work in them, and only peacekeepers are positioned as active agents), though there is an implicit suggestion that sex workers are likewise complicit in the spread of HIV. Female peacekeepers, unlikely to be patronizing "whorehouses", are likewise erased from view, resulting in the construction of peacekeepers and soldiers as an exclusively male population of autonomous sexual agents, able to control decisions about sexual activity including condom use. Underlying normative assumptions about peacekeepers' sexual behaviour thus enable a policy problem framing that obscures larger issues of gender, privilege, sexual agency, and the impact of peacekeeping missions on local economies, societies, and (predominantly female) bodies; and that overlooks structural, normative and other factors operating above the individual level to shape HIV risk (Phillips & Pirkle, 2011).

In sum, two narratives about HIV and security, each underpinned by very different normative assumptions and discourses, were driving HIV securitization efforts well before the UNSC sessions. Tension between these narratives would be evident in the sessions themselves, producing framing contests as actors debated the nature of the policy problem and threat posed by HIV, the appropriate referent object and meaning of security, and the threat responses that were therefore justified.

Persuasion, procedure and evidence in placing HIV on the UNSC agenda

Piot and Holbrooke (again, acting on behalf of larger constituencies) next sought to persuade other UN member states and actors in their own organizations that HIV was a security threat requiring UNSC consideration. In this second phase of their securitization efforts, tactics shifted from experiential approaches to rhetorical and procedural ones, including creative diplomacy and strategic use of evidence.

Creative diplomacy

Putting HIV on the UNSC agenda required creative interpretation of procedural rules, and negotiation to gain broader support. This charge was primarily led by Holbrooke, a seasoned diplomat and notoriously forceful personality. Holbrooke made innovative use of his presidency by declaring January 2000 'the month of Africa'. His invention of a thematic month at the UNSC, and use of this month to debate a non-traditional security issue, was both a procedural departure from usual UNSC practices and a political departure from the usual foreign policy preferences of the United States (Traub, 2006, p. 143). But while Holbrooke had considerable influence in setting the agenda, he also had to persuade sceptical UNSC permanent members that HIV was a suitable UNSC topic, or, at a minimum, persuade them not to block the discussion.[3] To secure the support of members who perceived HIV as an issue beyond UNSC responsibility, and better addressed by the ECOSOC agencies, a close advisor to Piot recalls that Holbrooke and his staff brokered an agreement with the P5 that the January 2000 debate would be a discussion only, and would not culminate in a resolution (Wayne, 2010). In the January UNSC session, then, concrete results in the form of a resolution were sacrificed in order to simply put HIV on the agenda.

The guarantee that there would be no resolution, and therefore no mechanism to hold states accountable for positions they expressed in the January session, may partly explain why many global North states felt free to initially make grand claims about human security, only to largely retreat from these when it came time to operationalize the UNSC response to HIV in a resolution. The resistance of the P5 to discussing HIV may also illuminate why HIV was initially framed as an *African* security threat. While the relationship between HIV and security was contested, security problems (in the most traditional sense) and HIV were each, as discussed in Chapter 3, already associated with Africa. Strategic deployment of the 'month of Africa' to justify discussion of HIV suggests that from the outset, Africa and its HIV pandemic were, in part, a means to an end, that end being less a conversation about HIV and Africa than about HIV and security, and ultimately, HIV and peacekeepers.

Creation, interpretation and use of evidence

Evidence was also used strategically in the lead-up to the debate to bolster support for the claim that HIV was a security threat. UNAIDS, under Piot's direction, began to compile evidence establishing the economic and security impact of HIV (Piot, 2009). These publications, often relying on limited epidemiological data described in alarming terms (Pisani, 2008, pp. 21–33), emphasized the magnitude of AIDS deaths, including that most HIV+ people "will die within a decade. These deaths will not be the last; there is worse to come" (Joint United Nations Programme on HIV/AIDS (UNAIDS), 1998b). They also claimed that HIV was impacting militaries and that war was a driver of HIV infection (Joint United Nations Programme on HIV/AIDS (UNAIDS), 1998a). Many of these findings were presented at global HIV/AIDS conferences, contributing, with the growing and vocal activist movement, to a general sense by the late 1990s that HIV was an urgent matter.

In the UN system, publications from international groups that had already begun to work with militaries on HIV were also circulating prior to the debate. These included papers written by the Civil Military Alliance to Combat HIV/

AIDS (CMA), an international alliance of military doctors, Surgeon Generals, and WHO staff in the Global Programme on AIDS (GPA), formed in 1995 to advocate for programmes to address HIV and/in militaries (Miller, January 1995) and UN peacekeeping (Boswell & Miller, January 1995), and for integration of civilian and military responses to HIV. Under CMA's auspices, work to address HIV in militaries and among peacekeepers was underway long prior to the UNSC debate (Geoff, 2009), much of it in tandem with GPA and later UNAIDS; the work included publications that represent some of the earliest international efforts to establish an evidence base linking HIV, militaries and peacekeeping (S. J. Kingma, 1996; Yeager, 1996).

The sense that HIV was a national security threat was further abetted by national-level analyses, many of them originating in the US, whose Department of Defense had also begun to develop HIV programmes for and with militaries, including in Africa, prior to 2000 (Ingram, 2011). These documents circulating in US foreign policy circles suggested that HIV contributed to state instability and conflict (Kaplan, 1994; National Intelligence Council, 2000; U.S. Department of State, 1995), that HIV rates were especially high in militaries due to soldiers' propensity for sexual risk-taking (U.S. Department of State, 1995), and therefore HIV rates among peacekeepers should be cause for concern (U.S. Department of State, 1995).

Overall this literature was not empirically well-supported – assertions about HIV and peacekeeping, in particular, had a very limited evidence base (Barnett & Prins, 2006; Elbe, 2009, pp. 27–58) – but was at the time widely accepted as credible. In contrast, there was ample evidence that new antiretroviral therapies were highly effective at prolonging the lives of PHAs. This evidence, while well-known and forming the basis for activist demands for universal treatment access, appears to have received less attention in the development of the evidence base that HIV was a security threat. Instead, efforts to link HIV and security focused on national security concerns including military prevalence rates, the sexual risk-taking of soldiers, and HIV as cause and consequence of armed conflict. This suggests that the initial securitizing actors either had deeply held assumptions that security 'really means' national security, or that they believed national security arguments would be more effective in the UN context. In either case, these seem to have encouraged strategic development of an HIV-and-security evidence narrative mainly reflecting national security concerns, in which the impact of AIDS-related deaths on states, not on people, is foregrounded.

This points to a notable silence in efforts to position HIV as a security threat and place it on the UNSC agenda: the voices of people living with HIV are almost entirely missing. Certainly some activists – to the extent that they were aware of manoeuvring to place HIV on the UNSC agenda – may have hoped that there would be instrumental use in this securitization, and that it might contribute to broader efforts to expand treatment access and end patent protections on ARVs. But many activists and PHAs were suspicious of securitizing moves. When asked how community-based activists responded to UNAIDS' use of security language, Piot recalled,

I think it was, in general, not always well-received, both positioning AIDS as an economic issue, or as a security issue. Because sometimes I was accused of.... "Isn't it bad enough, and isn't it a human rights issue?" And of course it is, I never forgot that or dropped it, but I was just trying to enlarge the audience, and the impact of what we do, and reaching people we don't reach. My obsession was to increase the money for AIDS. Not for UNAIDS, but for AIDS in developing countries, and two, to be able to provide treatment to people in developing countries.

(Piot, 2009)

Positioning HIV as a security problem was indeed effective at expanding the audience to include political leaders and military actors who had not been persuaded by human rights or social justice claims. But especially in the UNSC sessions, the goal of expanding treatment access, articulated through expansive human security claims, would sit in tension with earlier efforts to construct HIV as a security threat by linking HIV, conflict, militaries and state instability, which align more closely with national security concerns. And as we will see in the next chapter, it is far from clear that these security claims were more effective at increasing HIV funding than were other concurrent activist efforts.

Divergent agendas and framing contests: the Security Council debates HIV

The UNSC sessions mark the point at which prior successful securitizing strategies culminated in the speech acts at the core of HIV securitization. These speech acts include the sessions as a whole, statements made during the sessions, and Resolution 1308. Collectively, these constitute a securitizing speech act by CS standards (Buzan, Wæver, & de Wilde, 1998, esp. pp. 23–33 and 149): actors in structural positions of authority (the UNSC and ultimately all the P5) named HIV a security threat, as did several session participants, moving it into the UNSC realm of exceptional politics and signifying at least partial intersubjective agreement. The sessions broke the rule (the strong norm and UN Charter procedural guidelines) that the UNSC's area of concern is military threats to state security; by requiring subsequent DPKO action on HIV, Resolution 1308 broke the rule (again, the strong norm) that action on HIV should be led by health authorities; and resulting programming catalysed exceptional IO practices. These speech acts were not however straightforward declarations, but prolonged framing and meaning-making contests.

The UNSC held two sessions on HIV in 2000. The first was in January, where the agenda was "the impact of AIDS on peace and security in Africa". The session featured wide-ranging discussion about the impact of HIV on African people, states and institutions. The majority of speakers seemed initially to endorse an expansive human security vision in which the problem was human suffering, and the solution increased investments to support treatment access, reduction in drugs pricing and comprehensive HIV prevention, education, care and support. At the second session, in July, Africa dropped off the agenda, now "the responsibility of the Security Council in the maintenance of international peace and security: HIV/ AIDS and international peacekeeping operations". The debate ultimately entailed a policy frame informed by narrower national security concerns and focusing on the sexual behaviour of peacekeepers, and the proposed policy solution became HIV education and prevention programming for peacekeepers.

This was the directive ultimately entrenched in Resolution 1308. Pared down to a functional core, the response to the putative security threat posed by HIV ultimately entailed providing peacekeepers with condoms and HIV education. Yet it expanded the scope of UNSC authority significantly, to a scale at once much smaller (human bodies) and much larger (the world entire) than that at which it had previously operated: geographically bounded military conflicts. The resolution's preamble acknowledges "the severity of the crisis in Africa in particular" (United Nations Security Council, 17 July 2000), but its policy directive is HIV prevention programming for peacekeepers, not strategies to address the impact of the pandemic on the highest-prevalence sub-Saharan states. It makes only cursory reference to treatment, and does not acknowledge that a significant majority of people living with HIV in sub-Saharan Africa are women.

Framing the policy problem

Over the course of the UNSC sessions, multiple understandings of the relationship between HIV, Africa, peacekeeping and security were expressed. Participants debated the policy problem (is HIV a security threat? If so, how and to whom?) and the policy solution (what should be done?). Implicit in these framing contests were overarching debates about the meaning of security – especially whether it ought to be understood in narrow national security terms, privileging states and state sovereignty, or expansive human security terms, privileging the rights of populations over the sovereignty claims of states. Within this overarching national-or-human-security contest, policy problem framing further coalesced into debates about how Africa should be understood in relation to HIV and security, and how and to what extent peacekeepers were implicated. Policy solution disputes centred on the relative importance of HIV prevention education for peacekeepers, and investment in treatment access. The framing contests at the core of these securitizing speech acts therefore held deep normative and practical implications for the global response to HIV as well as international security.

National or human security?

All but two[4] of the 41 participants in the January UNSC session on "the impact of AIDS on peace and security in Africa" drew on the language and ideas of human security and national security to establish the relationship between HIV and Africa.[5] This affirms that actors' security speech in the UNSC, to be plausible and mutually intelligible, needed to conform to existing institutionalized definitions of security.

The majority of participants initially characterized HIV as a human security threat. Delegates explicitly used the term 'human security', spoke about the impact of HIV on individuals and communities, referred to human security principles such as protection from poverty and disease, and suggested that 'security' should be understood in broader terms. African and global South states in particular[6] (as well as the head of UNDP, the Ambassador for France, and Piot on behalf of UNAIDS), moved from invoking human security to advocating for increased treatment access and reallocation of resources:

> [I]n our view, security needs to be visualized as part of a complex of issues affecting the manner in which we perceive and deal with socioeconomic and political problems ... it is immoral that the worst-affected continent has the least access to the care and social and economic safety nets that might help families cope with the impact of this epidemic.
>
> (Dr. Amanthila, Namibia, United Nations Security Council, 2000b)

> HIV/AIDS threatens our security and our development. The country has already lost more than half a million people to this disease.... We lack resources. We are a poor country. Both the extended-family and government support systems are being overwhelmed by caring for orphans and the people living with AIDS. As the Council has already been told, the cost of providing anti-retroviral drugs is unaffordable in a country like ours and we do hope that the international community can come to our assistance in this respect.
>
> (Dr. Kiyonga, Uganda, United Nations Security Council, 2000b)

These claims discursively link HIV, especially and/in Africa, to a broader critique of health inequities, and make these the security problem to be addressed. On the one hand, invocations of human security entailed creative expression. As argued in the previous chapter, activist calls for treatment access were more usually expressed using critical social justice and structural violence analyses, but these held the latent potential to be expressed in human security terms. Delegates seized on this latent potential, attempting to fold activists' emancipatory claims into the language of human security that was intelligible as securitizing speech in the UNSC, and used this invocation of security to advocate for transformative ends.

But human security claims and calls for treatment access were intermingled, from the outset, with national security claims, pulling even seemingly expansive human security approaches back in the direction of narrower understandings of security. These national security claims included that AIDS deaths might threaten the stability, economic productivity and military preparedness of high-prevalence states:

> We know that poverty, hunger, debt and natural disasters, along with HIV/ AIDS, undermine African communities and destabilize African societies. This is likely to lead to the expansion of conflicts and crises.
>
> (Mustapha, Tunisia, in United Nations Security Council, 2000b)

The impact of AIDS on the countries of sub-Saharan Africa is especially devastating. It kills the most productive and active part of the population, thus increasing labour costs, reducing formal and informal sector productivity, eroding human, social, economic and infrastructure development and increasing health and welfare expenditures. AIDS also threatens the ability of African States to sustain credible defence forces, thus making it increasingly difficult to maintain domestic and regional security.

(Yel'chenko, Ukraine, in United Nations Security Council, 2000b)

Here, HIV and Africa are discursively linked to political instability and armed conflict. These claims align well with the evidence narrative strategically deployed prior to the debate in support of claims that HIV was a security problem because it threatened militaries and state stability; they also reflect and reinforce older discourses wherein Africa and HIV had already been produced as threatening to state and international system stability.

The shift from human to national security was also epitomized by the turn to peacekeeping in July 2000. As several delegates in the July session acknowledged, the turn in large part reflects bureaucratic context, in that peacekeeping is unambiguously a matter of UNSC authority in ways that HIV is not. But it is telling that the move from human to national security was also accomplished by discursively connecting peacekeepers to discourses in which Africans, soldiers and sex workers were already understood to be threats to national stability. Holbrooke's UNSC statements about peacekeepers, in particular, drew precisely on discourses in which unregulated African sexuality (specifically that of soldiers and sex workers) threatens order and stability.

Present and absent: the ambiguous status of Africa

The January 2000 session included wide-ranging discussion about HIV's impact on African political, economic and social life; yet some aspects of the discussion were facilitated by and further reinforced discourses constructing Africa as uniquely diseased, unstable, dangerous and therefore threatening. Throughout the debates, African and non-African participants alike struggled with this tension. Secretary-General Kofi Annan's statement exemplifies this struggle, and is worth quoting at length. He began by reciting dire statistics: 33 of the world's 48 least developed countries are in Africa; half of current armed conflicts are in Africa; 90% of the world's AIDS orphans are in Africa. But he then asserted that

there is no need to give way to Afro-pessimism. On the contrary, there could be no better moment for the international community to rally to Africa's support.... Some may say that [AIDS] should be left to other United Nations bodies. I believe, however, that the Council would not do itself justice if it held a month of Africa without discussing what Ambassador Holbrooke has called the number one problem facing Africa today. Not that AIDS is a purely African problem.... But nowhere else has AIDS yet become a threat to economic, social and political stability on the scale that it now is in southern and eastern Africa. The impact of AIDS in that region is no less destructive than that of warfare itself. Indeed, by some measures it is far worse. Last year, AIDS killed about 10 times more people in Africa than did armed conflict. By overwhelming the continent's health services, by creating millions of orphans and by decimating health workers and teachers, AIDS is causing social and economic crises, which in turn threaten political stability. It also threatens good governance through high death rates among the elites.... In already unstable societies, this cocktail of disasters is a sure recipe for more conflict, and conflict in turn provides fertile ground for further infections ... HIV/AIDS is not only an African problem. It is global and must be recognized as such. But within that international obligation the fight against AIDS in Africa is an immediate priority which must be part and parcel of our work for peace and security in that continent.

(Annan in United Nations Security Council, 2000b)

Annan moves from statistical evidence of Africa's challenges, to a renunciation of Afro-pessimism, back to a description of the crises and threats to stability that HIV is creating on the continent, then to an assertion that HIV is not an African but a global problem, then back again to the need to fight HIV in Africa in order to achieve peace and security there.

In suggesting that there is something special about the scope and impact of HIV *in Africa* that makes it a security challenge, both HIV exceptionalism and African exceptionalism are used to invoke another exceptionalism, that of securitization. Yet Annan simultaneously seeks to deny the exceptionalism this analysis suggests, namely that there is something uniquely threatening about HIV *in Africa*, by asserting, twice, that HIV is not an African but a global problem. In this denial is subtle recognition that there may be normative dangers in framing the security threat posed by HIV with reference to Africa. Reiterating this, Annan suggests that while HIV impact is borne disproportionately by Africans, this does not mean the *solution* is uniquely African: this is "a global problem" and addressing it an "international obligation".

Delegates also needed to engage in rhetorical contortion to make alleged links between HIV and conflict 'fit' the empirical reality of HIV prevalence across Africa. In specifying that HIV poses the greatest threat to stability in southern and eastern Africa (the regions with the highest HIV prevalence), Annan excludes north and west Africa (the latter in particular a region marked by considerable conflict and instability, and hosting the largest UN peace mission in 2000). Especially as the UNSC turned to peacekeeping, some delegates noted the contradiction between this focus and epidemiological data (detailed in Table 4.1) showing that HIV prevalence rates were highest in southern African states that were neither hosting, nor significant troop contributors to, peace missions. Indeed, the eventual reframing of HIV as a security threat in the context of peacekeeping served to exclude most of the African states and populations most affected by HIV. Of the approximately 29.5 million people living with HIV in

Table 4.1 HIV prevalence and UN peace missions

5 African states with highest HIV prevalence in 2001[1]	Hosting a peace mission?	Among top 5 troop contributing countries in January 2000?[2]	African states hosting peace missions in January 2000	State HIV prevalence rate, 2001	Top 5 African troop contributors, January 2000	State HIV prevalence rate, 2001
Botswana (26.5%)	No	No	**Sierra Leone**	1.3%	**Ghana**	2.3%
Swaziland (26.3%)	No	No	**Central African Republic**	6.4%	**Nigeria**	3.2%
Zimbabwe (26%)	No	No	**Western Sahara**	no data[3]	**Kenya**	no data
Lesotho (23.9%)	No	No	**Democratic Republic of the Congo**	no data	**Senegal**	0.4%
South Africa (16.9%)	No	No	**Angola**	1.6%	**Côte d'Ivoire**	6%

Notes

1 Data source for all HIV prevalence statistics in this table: *UNAIDS 2008 Report on the Global AIDS Epidemic*. These are estimates of adult (over age 15) prevalence in 2000, based on calculations completed in 2008.

2 These and all subsequent peacekeeping data in Tables 4.2 and 4.3 are from the UN Peacekeeping Monthly Summary of Contributors of Military and Civilian Police Personnel archives, available on the Department of Peacekeeping Operations' website: www.un.org/en/peacekeeping/resources/statistics/contributors_archive.shtml (accessed 30 October 2013). Numbers include troops, police, and uniformed service observers.

3 For regions with no data, in 2012 there continued to be no data for Western Sahara. UNAIDS' estimated adult (age 15–49) prevalence was 1.1% for the Democratic Republic of the Congo (www.unaids.org/en/regionscountries/countries/democraticrepublicofthecongo/, accessed October 30, 2013) and 6.1% for Kenya (www.unaids.org/en/regionscountries/countries/kenya/, accessed October 30, 2013).

2001, 20.4 million were in sub-Saharan Africa (Joint United Nations Programme on HIV/AIDS (UNAIDS), 2008, p. 214),[7] but these were not, for the most part, the continent's least stable regions or the hosts of peacekeeping missions. Furthermore, more than half of sub-Saharan Africa's HIV-positive population were women (Joint United Nations Programme on HIV/AIDS (UNAIDS), 2008, p. 216), whereas peacekeepers are a predominantly male population.

Africa, having been invoked in the initial move to securitize HIV, became less visible in the July UNSC session, where the focus narrowed from potentially the entire population of Africa to fewer than 20,000 peacekeepers. Though the turn to peacekeepers in one sense constituted a dramatic shift away from Africa, in fact the continent became not absent but hidden. In 2000 Africa was home to three of the top ten troop contributing countries (see Table 4.2) and five of 19 peacekeeping missions, including the then-largest mission in Sierra Leone (see Table 4.3); these states remained deeply implicated in any discussions about peacekeeping by virtue of their status as troop contributing and receiving countries.

Strategic deployment of narratives about Africa and security, in which HIV was only one of a broader constellation of security challenges on the continent,

Table 4.2 Top UN troop contributors in 2000

Top 10 troop contributors, January 2000	*Number of uniformed services deployed*
India	2,297 (26 observer, 224 police, 2,047 troop)
Ghana	**1,701** **(18 observer, 243 police, 1,440 troop)**
Nigeria	**1,616** **(17 observer, 38 police, 1,561 troop)**
Poland	1,060 (19 observer, 57 police, 984 troop)
Bangladesh	944 (69 observer, 69 police, 806 troop)
Kenya	**886** **(26 observer, 28 police, 832 troop)**
Austria	723 (26 observer, 91 police, 606 troop)
Argentina	703 (10 observer, 203 police, 490 troop)
Ireland	688 (30 observer, 48 police, 610 troop)
USA	653 (32 observer, 621 police, 0 troop)
Total **Total African**	11,271 **4,203 (37% of gross total)**

Table 4.3 African deployment in UN peace missions in 2000

Military and CivPol deployment by mission, c.2000 (African missions in bold)

Mission	Total deployment	Total deployed from African states (includes Egypt)
UNAMSIL (Sierra Leone)	**4,848 (243 observer, 4 police, 4601 troop)**	**3,255 (67%)**
UNIFIL (Lebanon)	4,495 (4,495 troop)	900 (20%)
UNMIK (Kosovo)	2,006 (35 observer, 1971 police, 0 troop)	232 (11.5%)
UNMIBH (Bosnia & Herzegovina)	1,746 (4 observer, 1742 police, 0 troop)	290 (17%)
UNFICYP (Cyprus)	1,250 (0 observer, 33 police, 1217 troop)	0
UNIKOM (Iraq & Kuwait)	1,093 (194 observer, 0 police, 899 troop)	19 (2%)
UNDOF (Golan Heights)	1,037 (1037 troop)	0
UNTAET (East Timor)	669 (184 observer, 481 police, 4 troop)	206 (31%)
MINURCA (Central African Republic)	**438 (0 observer, 9 police, 429 troop)**	**334 (76%)**
MINURSO (Western Sahara)	**310 (204 observer, 79 police, 27 troop)**	**72 (23%)**
MIPONUH (Haiti)	241 (241 police)	0
UNTSO (Middle East)	152 (152 observer)	0
UNOMIG (Georgia)	101 (101 observer)	6 (6%)
MONUC (DRC)	**79 (79 observer)**	**31 (39%)**
MINUGUA (Guatemala)	70 (20 observer, 50 police, 0 troop)	0
UNMOGIP (India & Pakistan)	46 (46 observer)	0
UNMOT (Tajikistan)	32 (30 observer, 2 police)	9 (28%)
UNMOP (Croatia & Yugoslavia)	27 (27 observer)	5 (18.5%)
MONUA (Angola)	**3 (1 observer, 1 police, 1 troop)**	**1 (33%)**
	Total deployed worldwide 18,643 Total deployed *in* African states: 5,678 (30% of total deployment)	Total deployed *from* African states: 5,360 (29% of total deployment)

was used to justify placing HIV on the UNSC agenda. But from the outset, the reality of HIV's impact in Africa sat in tension with narratives about the interplay between HIV, conflict and peacekeeping. It is an example of the ways that "narrative about Africa is always a pretext for a comment about something else, some other place, some other people" (Mbembe, 2001, pp. 2–3). In this case, narrative about the impact of HIV in Africa facilitated forms of threat construction, and the production of an HIV securitization, ultimately not directed towards addressing the African HIV pandemic.

Threatened or threatening? The dual status of peacekeepers

Most debate participants were less certain than Holbrooke of the extent to which HIV and peacekeeping were related, and if they were, whether peacekeepers themselves were threats, or were threatened by HIV. Consistent with the HIV discourses explored in the previous chapter, that work to produce binary categories of innocent victims and morally culpable and dangerous vectors of disease, the same pattern emerges in UNSC discussions about peacekeepers.

Three possible linkages between HIV and peacekeeping were suggested. First, peacekeepers were imagined as threatened by HIV. US Vice President Al Gore, for example, suggested that HIV in sub-Saharan Africa "is a security crisis, because it threatens not only individual citizens but the institutions that define and defend the character of a society.... It strikes at the military and subverts the forces of order and peacekeeping" (Gore in United Nations Security Council, 2000b). Here, peacekeepers and the institution of peacekeeping are constructed as threatened by HIV because of high rates of HIV in the militaries of sub-Saharan states. Notably, this construction also dovetails with discourses about Africa in which the continent is constructed as dangerously unstable, and with national security concerns for order, stability and military integrity.

Second, peacekeepers were imagined as threatening vectors, with Holbrooke insisting, "it is a fact that without proper training, education and steps towards prevention, peacekeepers may also be spreading AIDS inadvertently" (Holbrooke in United Nations Security Council, 2000a). Other delegates, linking HIV, peacekeeping, and conflict, observed that rape and sexual violence perpetrated by uniformed services members could spread HIV. The implication was that soldiers, including peacekeepers, might be dangerous not just as HIV vectors, but also perpetrators of sexual abuse. It is an implication borne out by revelations around the same time as the UNSC sessions of peacekeepers' involvement in sexual exploitation and abuse; this triggered the creation in 2000 of a DPKO unit devoted to preventing and prosecuting sexual abuse in peacekeeping missions.

These two policy problem frames exemplify the tendency of securitization to, via threat construction, produce binary categories of threatened and threatening subjects. While debate participants advancing these frames disagreed about whether peacekeepers were threatened or threatening, both perspectives follow securitization's binary logic. There was however a third, minority position expressed. Piot contended that "[h]umanitarian aid workers and military and police forces that are well trained in HIV prevention and behaviour change can be a tremendous force for prevention as long as this is made one of their priorities" (Piot in United Nations Security Council, 2000b), while the Tunisian delegate suggested "peacekeeping forces can play an important role in awareness-raising and providing a means of prevention for themselves and others" (Ben Mustapha in United Nations Security Council, 2000a). This counter-narrative, attempting to break out of binary threatened/threatening subject categories by imagining a new identity in which peacekeepers are educators, is another instance of actors seeking creative potential in and against securitization logic. At the initial policy framing and implementation stage, the other two constructions of peacekeepers dominated, but as shown in Chapter 6, this counter-narrative would work quietly in the background and re-emerge over the next decade.

Framing the policy solution: prevention for peacekeepers or treatment for all?

For high-prevalence states, the overwhelming problem posed by HIV was lack of treatment access, largely due to prohibitively high ARV prices. Conveying the magnitude of this challenge, the Ugandan health minister explained that

> [u]nder the drug-access programme sponsored by [UNAIDS] ... only about 1,000 Ugandans have benefited from HIV/AIDS anti-retroviral treatment. This is mainly due to the high cost of drugs ... a monthly supply of drugs costs about $12,000 per patient per year. With the estimated 2 million Ugandans infected with HIV, universal access would cost us $24 billion. This is in contrast to our annual budget of $2 billion.
>
> (Kiyonga in United Nations Security Council, 2000b)

The policy solution for these delegates was obviously improved treatment access, especially in the highest-prevalence states in southern Africa, as

> prevention alone is not sufficient, given the large numbers of people already infected with the virus. Due to a lack of resources and the inaccessibility of HIV drugs, not much progress has been attained in the treatment of the disease. Thus, Governments cannot do much for the people already infected, who are therefore left to die without hope of treatment.
>
> (Andjaba, Namibia, in United Nations Security Council, 2000a)

Compelling pharmaceutical companies to reduce drug prices was repeatedly suggested as one measure that should be taken, along with increased financial commitments.

Yet the July 2000 UNSC session turned away from the issue of treatment access, reframing the policy problem as HIV in peacekeeping. While delegates acknowledged that effectively addressing HIV required significant action to improve access to HIV education, prevention and treatment, most global North delegates suggested that this was simply beyond the authority of the UNSC, and spoke approvingly of the UNSC's decision to address HIV exclusively within UN peacekeepers. The majority of speakers appeared to accept that peacekeepers were vulnerable to HIV, might be inadvertently spreading it, and were in need of HIV education – and that this, after months of deliberation and two UNSC sessions devoted to HIV, was the most appropriate intervention for the UNSC to make in the global response.

It was a disappointing outcome for at least some of the African states addressing the UNSC, who continued to advocate for treatment access. The delegate from Malawi, whose country had deployed only one peacekeeper in 2000 but had an estimated adult HIV prevalence rate of 13% (Joint United Nations Programme on HIV/AIDS (UNAIDS), 2008, p. 215), epitomized this frustration, stating:

> The Malawian delegation believed that the Security Council discussions in January might produce fresh ideas for combating AIDS, because it should have been clear to all involved that the strategies that had theretofore been adopted to combat HIV infection had failed. Unfortunately, this was not to be. What emerged was a reinforcement of the same old strategies, with perhaps a little more vigour this time around.
>
> (Juwayeyi in United Nations Security Council, 2000a)

The difficulty with the ultimate focus on prevention for peacekeepers was twofold. First, as the Malawian delegate recognized, it hardly constituted a meaningful response to HIV; the vast majority of people living with and vulnerable to HIV are neither peacekeepers nor their sexual partners. Second, HIV education programming with militaries was *already* underway both in and beyond the UN well before 2000, including through the Civil–Military Alliance to Combat HIV/AIDS, GPA and UNFPA programming, and bilateral US Department of Defense programmes. As a response to the policy problem as originally stated, that HIV was a security threat to and in Africa, the prevention- and peacekeeper-focused Resolution 1308 was hardly a robust response.

The stakes in these framing contests are significant. When HIV is seen as a (mainly national security) threat because of the sexual practices of individual soldiers or peacekeepers, the policy solution becomes education and individual behaviour change interventions. But when the policy problem is economic and political barriers to treatment access, the policy solution is understood as structural reform to address health inequities. In other words, the pandemic is framed as a problem with largely structural origins and solutions; it is the socio-economic conditions under which HIV transmission occurs that are foregrounded, and far-reaching economic and political reforms are indicated. In contrast, when the security threat posed by HIV is understood as a problem of individual peacekeepers' sexual behaviour, the policy solution need be no more radical than the status quo, plus condoms.

The impact of securitization logic

The direct result of the UNSC session was that some populations (peacekeepers and to a lesser extent their sexual partners) and some territories (sites of peace-keeping and armed conflict) were securitized as threats. Expansive arguments for investments to support universal treatment access failed, in the end, to gain traction in the UNSC, with the result that the people and places most affected by HIV remained outside of the UNSC's HIV securitization.

One explanation for this outcome is that structurally powerful global North states were protecting their economic interests, and their behaviour was a predictable consequence of realist power politics. Certainly it would be naïve to suggest that these political and economic factors were not at work. But these same states would very shortly commit significant new funds to HIV, and support reductions in drug pricing and sales of generic ARVs, against the wishes of pharmaceutical firms attempting to defend their patent rights. Demands that global North states support significant resource reallocation and market transformation (Kapstein & Busby, 2013), that is, were highly successful elsewhere in the global response. They just were not successful in the context of the UNSC, and in the context of securitization strategies.

The organizational context of the UNSC clearly influenced the contours of HIV securitization and contributed to the narrowing of policy problem and solution frames. Security has a specific and circumscribed meaning in the UN, which meant that from the outset the available definitions of security were national and human security. Furthermore, the UNSC needed to respond to HIV in a manner consistent with its scope of authority and mandate to safeguard international peace and security (Rushton, 2010), which meant that peacekeepers were among the only populations over whom the UNSC could exercise significant authority. Finally, the slippage in the UNSC sessions from security to the security sector to peacekeepers reflects that empirically, notwithstanding the circulation of human security discourses, security and therefore activities designated as security-related are, in most of the UN system, equated to work with and in the security sector, defined as militaries and other uniformed services, and conflict and post-conflict territories. (This empirical conflation of security and the security sector in the UN system is explored in the next chapter's discussion of the boundary work undertaken to maintain this meaning of security.) The UNSC itself, then, may not be an especially effective site for securitization strategies primarily intended to produce change outside the realm of the security sector.

The formally narrow outcome of the UNSC sessions was in part a product of features of the UN system. But the logic of threat construction and response that animated policy problem and solution framing contests also held inherent constraints; these are due not to the location of securitization efforts but to the logic of securitization itself. In particular, the logic of securitization required HIV to be cast as a security *threat*. This can be (and ultimately was) most effectively accomplished through explicitly threat-based discourses in which HIV, Africa and 'high risk' populations, including soldiers and sex workers, are constructed as threats, while the referent objects are non-African people and states, as well as international stability and systems writ large. These are more congruent with the national security concerns which in turn supported the successful, narrowly defined policy problem and solution frames.

Threat constructions, with their binary inside/outside, threatened/threatening, us/Other categories, were present from the first securitizing strategies, when Holbrooke's visit to Africa led him to imagine threatened victims who would "get" HIV and threatening vectors who would "spread" it. Securitization's logic of binary threat construction recurred throughout the UNSC sessions, especially in framing debates about whether peacekeepers were threatened or threatening. They were also evident (though usually implicit rather than overt) in the threat-based discourses about Africa and HIV that facilitated the initial securitizing move, and then undergirded the turn to peacekeeping. The tendency of securitization's threat constructions to then produce defensive threat response is finally evident in Resolution 1308's policy directive calling for HIV prevention programmes and condoms for peacekeepers. This is a defensive move entailing threat containment and literal prophylaxis against threatening Others, in which peacekeepers, reduced to vectors, become a source of contagion to be contained.

Conclusion

This chapter has argued that the strategies, speech acts and framing contests that placed HIV on the UNSC agenda and culminated in Resolution 1308 were, from the outset, characterized by tensions and contradictions. Securitization efforts entailed creative strategies to bring HIV to the UNSC, creative efforts to rearticulate, in human security terms, the need for treatment access and transformation in the global response, and significant meaning-making contests as participants advanced different understandings of how and to whom HIV might be a security threat. But these were constrained by organizational features of the UN system, and by securitization's logic of threat construction and response. As the human security problem of HIV in Africa was reframed into a national security problem of HIV in peacekeeping, despite attempts to advance counter-narratives in support of treatment access, the UNSC sessions produced an outcome that did not meaningfully address the impact of HIV in Africa. Against the transformative aims of at least some participants, a narrower narrative of and policy response to peacekeepers as HIV threats won out.

The analysis already begins to suggest some limitations to securitization as a social justice strategy. The gravitational pull exerted by national security in the UNSC sessions, while certainly indicating the effect of context in shaping securitization, is also suggestive of strongly held beliefs about what security 'really means'. Even UNAIDS, in developing evidence to connect HIV and security with the intent to catalyse transformation of the global response, tacitly accepted a mainly national security understanding of security as referring to militaries, armed conflict, and state stability. Debate participants who challenged this understanding, calling instead for expansive human security approaches, were ultimately unsuccessful in dislodging the dominant UNSC understanding of security as national security. This empirical outcome may lend further weight to critiques of human security that suggest it operates mainly within, rather than representing a significant departure from, dominant security logics (Chandler, 2008; Rushton, 2011; Seckinelgin, 2012, pp. 181–182). The seemingly deeply entrenched meaning of security-in-use may additionally suggest limits to what security, not just securitization, can be made to do in practice, at least in the organizational context of the UN. This need not become an argument against the constructed nature of security in principle, but it is certainly a cautionary observation about its empirical limits in practice.

The assessment that the UNSC sessions' outcome was limited relative to the ambitions of some of the UNSC session architects, and to the initial agenda to address HIV's impact on peace and security in Africa, does not mean the sessions had no impact. They clearly held symbolic value, signifying that states, including powerful UN donor states, were beginning to take HIV seriously as a matter requiring coordinated global response. This served to increase UNAIDS' legitimacy and authority, as it now had the weight of the UNSC and its permanent members behind its work, and high-level recognition of that work as a political priority. Piot recalls that the UNSC sessions and Resolution 1308, by providing this political legitimacy and authority, consequently "opened so many doors" (Piot, 2009) for UNAIDS. Further, as discussed in the next chapter, Resolution 1308 would have significant impact within the UN's resulting 'security response' to HIV, even if it had little impact on the larger global response. The aim of the analysis has been, therefore, to discover how securitization worked in and through framing contests to produce this outcome.

Finally, this should not be read as a fatalistic or deterministic analysis. Securitization logic, while producing strong constraints, was not absolute, as evident from some UNSC session participants' efforts to work creatively in and against this logic to articulate alternative policy problem and solution frames. While Resolution 1308 was unanimously adopted, there remained little consensus about the relationship between HIV, security and peacekeeping, and there continued to be latent possibilities for different interpretations that could be – and, as shown in the next chapter, ultimately were – exploited at the policy implementation stage as HIV securitization moved out of the UNSC and into the wider UN bureaucracy.

Notes

1 Some sections of this chapter are adapted from a working paper (Hindmarch, 2008).
2 This strategy, and securitizing logic, of pursuing a high-level directive to circumvent bureaucratic politicking was likely also a response to "constant, never-ending friction with the [UNAIDS] cosponsoring agencies" in the early years of UNAIDS (Piot, 2012).
3 China, France (Prins, 2004, p. 941), the Russian Federation (Sternberg, 2002), and the UK (McInnes & Rushton, 2010, p. 230, note 23) were all initially resistant to discussing HIV in the UNSC.

4 These were Cuba and Zimbabwe. Only Cuba directly challenged the idea that HIV is a security threat, stating "AIDS in Africa, like hunger, is a problem of underdevelopment, not of security" (Rodriguez Parrilla in United Nations Security Council, 2000b).

5 Transcripts of the 10 January 2000 UNSC session were analysed for national security content (referent object is states, bounded territories, economic systems, political systems, military and/or peacekeeping capabilities; reference to protection from disease as a means of securing power resources such as economies, agricultural or industrial development and protecting political, economic and social order and stability) or human security content (referent object is people or communities, including global community and specific populations; references to broadening/widening/deepening security or to non-traditional security threats; protection from disease as a means of promoting human well-being). Each speaker's contribution was coded as primarily national security; primarily human security; both national and human security; neither national nor human security. Thirty-two speakers discussed HIV in human security terms, and 28 in national security terms (numbers add up to more than the 41 unique participants because several speakers positioned HIV as both a human and national security threat).

6 Fourteen of the 37 speakers in the January debate were African delegates, reflecting the importance of the session to African states. Namibia, Uganda and Zimbabwe sent their health ministers (i.e. senior political officials) rather than their ambassadors, further signifying the importance of the session to these states.

7 These and subsequent HIV statistics are from 2001 because it is the closest year to the UNSC debate for which there is a complete data set. These estimates were retroactively revised downwards by UNAIDS and WHO in December 2007, and so are slightly lower (29 million rather than 32 million) than the global incidence estimates available to delegates at the time of the debate. The 29.5 million figure includes all ages and genders.

References

Barnett, T. & Prins, G. (2006). HIV/AIDS and security: fact, fiction and evidence – a report to UNAIDS. *International Affairs, 82*(2), 359–368.

Boswell, R. N. & Miller, N. (January 1995). New international organization responds to HIV/AIDS challenge. *Civil–Military Alliance Newsletter, 1*(1), 1.

Buzan, B., Wæver, O., & de Wilde, J. (1998). *Security: A New Framework for Analysis.* Boulder, CO: Lynne Rienner.

Chandler, D. (2008). Human security: the dog that didn't bark. *Security Dialogue, 39*(4), 427–438.

David, M. (2001). Rubber helmets: the certain pitfalls of marshalling Security Council resources to combat AIDS in Africa. *Human Rights Quarterly, 23*(3), 560–582.

Elbe, S. (2009). *Virus Alert: Security, Governmentality, and the AIDS Pandemic.* New York: Columbia University Press.

Geoff. (2009, 17 December). (Personal interview with author).

Hindmarch, S. (2008). The implications of treating HIV as a security threat in Africa: an analysis of the United Nations Security Council debate on HIV. In S. Allin & M. B. Seaton (Eds.), *Comparative Program on Health and Society Lupina Foundation Working Papers Series 2007–09* (pp. 76–97). Toronto: Munk Centre for International Studies (MCIS Briefings).

Ingram, A. (2011). The Pentagon's HIV/AIDS programmes: governmentality, political economy, security. *Geopolitics, 16*(3), 655–674.

Ingram, A. (2013). After the exception: HIV/AIDS beyond salvation and scarcity. *Antipode*, *45*(2), 436–454.

Joint United Nations Programme on HIV/AIDS (UNAIDS). (1998a). AIDS and the military: UNAIDS point of view. Geneva: UNAIDS.

Joint United Nations Programme on HIV/AIDS (UNAIDS). (1998b). Report on the global HIV/AIDS epidemic. Geneva: UNAIDS.

Joint United Nations Programme on HIV/AIDS (UNAIDS). (2008). 2008 Report on the global AIDS epidemic. Geneva: Joint United Nations Programme on HIV/AIDS (UNAIDS).

Kaplan, R. D. (1994). The coming anarchy. *The Atlantic Monthly*, *273*(2), 44–76.

Kapstein, E. B. & Busby, J. W. (2013). *AIDS Drugs for All: Social Movements and Market Transformations*. Cambridge, UK: Cambridge University Press.

Kingma, S. J. (1996). *Occasional Paper Series No. 2: AIDS Prevention in Military Populations: Learning the Lessons of History*. Geneva: Civil–Military Alliance to Combat HIV and AIDS.

Knight, L. (2008). *UNAIDS: The First 10 Years, 1996–2006*. Geneva: Joint United Nations Programme on HIV/AIDS (UNAIDS).

Mbembe, A. (2001). *On the Postcolony* (A. M. Berrett, J. Roitman, M. Last, & S. Rendall, Trans.). Berkeley, CA: University of California Press.

McInnes, C. & Rushton, S. (2010). HIV, AIDS and security: where are we now? *International Affairs*, *86*(1), 225–245.

McInnes, C. & Rushton, S. (2013). HIV/AIDS and securitization theory. *European Journal of International Relations*, *19*(1), 115–138.

Miller, N. (January 1995). Alliance: the issues at stake. *Civil–Military Alliance Newsletter*, *1*(1), 2.

National Intelligence Council. (2000). The global infectious disease threat and its implications for the United States. Langley: National Intelligence Council.

PBS. (2006, 30 May). Interview, Richard Holbrooke. *Frontline: The Age of AIDS* Retrieved 24 June 2011 from www.pbs.org/wgbh/pages/frontline/aids/interviews/holbrooke.html#ixzz1QJr3Zjvl.

Phillips, A. F. & Pirkle, C. M. (2011). Moving beyond behaviour: advancing HIV risk prevention epistemologies (a report on the state of the literature). *Global Public Health*, *6*(6), 577–592.

Piot, P. (2009, 23 October). (Personal interview with author.)

Pisani, E. (2008). *The Wisdom of Whores: Bureaucrats, Brothels and the Business of AIDS*. Toronto: Penguin Group (Canada).

Prins, G. (2004). AIDS and global security. *International Affairs*, *80*(5), 931–952.

Rushton, S. (2010). Framing AIDS: securitization, development-ization, rights-ization. *Global Health Governance*, *4*(2), 1–17.

Rushton, S. (2011). Global health security: security for whom? Security from what? *Political Studies*, *59*(4), 779–796.

Seckinelgin, H. (2012). *International Security, Conflict and Gender: "HIV/AIDS Is Another War"*. New York: Routledge.

Sjöstedt, R. (2011). Health issues and securitization: the construction of HIV/AIDS as a US national security threat. In T. Balzacq (Ed.), *Securitization Theory: How Security Problems Emerge and Dissolve* (pp. 150–169). New York: Routledge.

Stein, G. (1960 [1933]). *The Autobiography of Alice B. Toklas*. New York: Vintage Books.

Sternberg, S. (2002, 11 June). The Fixer takes on global AIDS; Richard Holbrooke faces the biggest challenge of his storied career. *USA Today*, D07.

Traub, J. (2006). *The Best Intentions: Kofi Annan and the UN in the Era of American World Power*. New York: Farrar, Straus and Giroux.

U.S. Department of State. (1995). U.S. International strategy on HIV/AIDS. Retrieved 8 November 2012 from http://dosfan.lib.uic.edu/ERC/environment/releases/9507.html.

United Nations Security Council. (17 July 2000). Resolution 1308 (2000) (S/RES/1308(2000) – adopted by the Security Council at its 4172nd meeting, 17 July 2000).

United Nations Security Council. (2000a). Transcript: Agenda: The responsibility of the Security Council in the maintenance of international peace and security: HIV/AIDS and international peacekeeping operations (Security Council 55th year, 4172nd meeting, Monday 17 July 2000 S/PV.4172).

United Nations Security Council. (2000b). Transcript: Agenda: The situation in Africa: the impact of AIDS on peace and security in Africa (Security Council 55th year, 4087 meeting, Monday 10 January 2000 S/PV.4087 (Resumption 1)).

Wayne (2010, 13 April). (Personal interview with author.)

Yeager, R. (1996). *Occasional Paper Series No. 1: Military HIV/AIDS Policy in Eastern and Southern Africa: A Seven-Country Comparison*. Geneva: Civil–Military Alliance to Combat HIV and AIDS.

5 When urgency meets bureaucracy

Boundary work in HIV and security policy implementation

Resolution 1308 provided UN staff with a high-level policy directive, but translating this directive into programmes and practices was a contested interpretive process. At the implementation stage, the ideas about HIV and security that had been articulated in the UNSC sessions collided with entrenched bureaucratic practices, and with bureaucratic actors' own ideas about HIV, health and security, which at times differed significantly from those of the original architects of HIV securitization. What then happened when urgency met bureaucracy: when the securitized response to HIV, embodied in the ideas and policy directives expressed in UNSC sessions and Resolution 1308, met UN organizational structures, norms and practices?

This chapter demonstrates that the policy implementation process following Resolution 1308 involved ongoing contestations about HIV and security, both as an idea and a set of bureaucratic practices in the UN system. The formally narrow mandate of Resolution 1308 initially resulted in similarly narrow programming, that is, basic HIV education for peacekeepers. This programming, though restricted to the security sector, broadened and deepened over time as actors introduced more diverse and far-reaching interventions with uniformed services. Yet these programming interventions and accompanying normative debates, refracted through the lens of security, often took on a significantly different tone and form than those in community-based responses to HIV.

The chapter begins with an overview of organizational and funding changes in the global response to HIV, within and beyond the UN, after 2000. It shows that Resolution 1308 was directly responsible for some minor restructuring in UNAIDS, and for new programming for peacekeepers, but that the most significant transformations in the global response in this period occurred outside of UNSC-centred securitization efforts. However, HIV securitization, particularly Resolution 1308, had significant albeit localized consequences. These are explored in the chapter's second section, which explores the normative contests that occurred as Resolution 1308 was implemented. These contestations coalesced around two interpretive disputes, each involving 'boundary work' (Gieryn, 1983) by bureaucratic actors. The first dispute was about the *categorization* of HIV and security programming, including the meaning and borders of 'security' activities in the UN. Here, long-standing normative and jurisdictional tensions between humanitarian and security actors in the UN became newly salient. The second involved the *content* of HIV and security programming, and focused on questions about the proper extent and reach of programming in the emerging 'security response' to HIV. Through these disputes, actors renegotiated responsibilities, activities and spheres of authority in ways that ultimately expanded the authority of some UN actors and produced deeper incursions into some states and bodies. At the same time, boundary work further entrenched actors' already-existing beliefs about what security 'really means', and which activities can properly be undertaken in programming designated as security-related. The chapter concludes by drawing out the consequences of this meeting of urgency and bureaucracy, and of security and health: that the logic of securitization, in conjunction with boundary work undertaken to maintain organizational definitions of security, served to privilege the sovereignty and autonomy of some states and bodies, support transgression into others, all while placing some of the people and places most affected by HIV entirely outside of this securitized response.

The analysis focuses specifically on UN peacekeeping, reflecting that empirically, as shown in Chapter 4, securitizing actors themselves immediately conflated security with the security sector. While securitization theory is mainly interested in the grammar, logic and effects of securitization, not the word 'security' (Buzan, Wæver, & de Wilde, 1998), in practice HIV securitization entailed quite explicit focus on, and assumptions about, the meaning of the word 'security', and these assumptions significantly influenced how the grammar and logic of the securitizing speech act were interpreted and implemented. Put differently, the deeply engrained belief that security refers to the security sector is also evident in the wider UN bureaucracy, where Resolution 1308 is understood to have produced the 'security response to HIV', which is for these bureaucratic actors synonymous with HIV programming in and for the security sector, particularly with UN peacekeepers.

Changes in the global response after 2000: what did Resolution 1308 do, and not do?

It has by now been well-established that the most consequential events in the global response around 2000 – changes to patent protections and pricing of ARVs – resulted from concerted, coordinated civil society activism (Gray, 2012; Kapstein & Busby, 2013; Smith & Siplon, 2006). The UNSC sessions were mainly a symptom, not a cause, of this larger movement. While holding some symbolic value, there is no evidence that the UNSC sessions were in any meaningful sense responsible for the improvement in treatment access catalysed by this unprecedented civil society mobilization. To further untangle the direct impact of Resolution 1308 and the UNSC sessions from events in the broader global response, two additional empirical indicators can be considered. First, we can assess financial impact, comparing HIV and security spending to new investments in the global response writ large; second, we can assess the extent to which Resolution 1308 catalysed organizational change in the UN system.

Global HIV spending after 2000

Global HIV funding allocations increased significantly after 2000 due to a number of large multilateral initiatives.[1] These included the Global Fund to Fight AIDS, Tuberculosis and Malaria (the Global Fund), created in January 2002. The Global Fund has a budget far larger than UNAIDS and most other multilateral actors, and larger than the GDP of many of the countries in which it operates (The Global Fund to Fight AIDS, Tuberculosis and Malaria, 2002, 2012).

Although negotiations to establish the Global Fund coincided with efforts to place HIV on the UNSC agenda, there is little evidence to suggest that security concerns in general, or the UNSC sessions in particular, were the impetus for the fund's creation. Global Fund literature does not describe HIV as a security problem or invoke security rhetoric in describing its work. Furthermore, two highly-placed interviewees involved in Global Fund negotiations did not recall security concerns or securitizing logic being invoked in formal closed-door sessions or informal 'corridor chats' that preceded the Fund's creation:

> We found the security argument very difficult to put forward as a compelling driver of action against AIDS.... We found better economic arguments.... [W]e felt that the economic argument was an easier argument for ordinary people as well as most decision-makers to wrap their heads around, because the security argument was so apocalyptic in nature that it seemed harder for people to really relate to.
>
> (Senior advisor to WHO leadership – Patrick, 2009)

> STEPHEN LEWIS (SL): I was in on all the early discussions of the Global Fund ...I was the Envoy, so I would meet with Kofi Annan and Richard Feachem [Global Fund director].... *Never*, in those early discussions as the Global Fund was getting off the ground do I remember security having been mentioned.
>
> SH: How do you remember it being discussed?
>
> SL: Oh, just as a health issue, yeah, also as a humanitarian issue. By that time people were beginning to see that it had social and economic implications that went way beyond the provision of treatment, but don't forget that the driving force ... was treatment. That was the issue. Security had nothing to do with it.
>
> (Lewis, 2011)

Both of these interviewees maintained that what drove the creation of the Global Fund was concern about the poverty and development impact of HIV – an impact that did not, for Global Fund architects, need to be recast in security terms to justify urgent action. In sum, while there was a significant increase in HIV funding in the global response writ large after 2000, this appears to have occurred in parallel with but largely separate from securitization efforts (McInnes & Rushton have reached similar conclusions: see McInnes & Rushton, 2010, 2013; Rushton, 2010a).

Indeed, in spite of new investments in HIV after 2000, funds for the security response to HIV remained limited – suggesting that UNSC-based securitization efforts had limited success in leveraging significant new donor funds for HIV and security-specific programming. By 2003 the DPKO had established a small fund of a few hundred thousand dollars for prevention education (Joint United Nations Programme on HIV/AIDS (UNAIDS), 2003b, p. 4; 2004, p. 13). But DPKO staff working on HIV programming for peacekeepers still regard available funds as inadequate: "because HIV is not the core business of peacekeeping, naturally we are not given all that we need, and we have to do with resources which are actually quite constrained" (Alex, 2010).

It is perhaps unsurprising that DPKO spending on HIV remained limited after Resolution 1308, since the success of peacekeeping missions is far more dependent on other factors. But even in UNAIDS, where we might expect to see a more significant investment in the security response to HIV, funds remained limited. Peter Piot (2009) recalled that following Resolution 1308, "we didn't have the resources to develop this [HIV and security programmes] into a big thing. We were dependent on the individual donor contributions". In 2004, UNAIDS committed just over US$1.9 million for uniformed services HIV education programming, which was disbursed in smaller amounts to country-specific projects (Joint United Nations Programme on HIV/AIDS (UNAIDS), 2004). These expenditures represent a small fraction of the overall budget for UNAIDS. While the total UNAIDS budget increased significantly after 2000, this was mainly due to an unrelated administrative change in UN budget and workplan development (UNAIDS Programme Coordinating Board, 2002, p. x).[2]

Staff in other UN agencies also noted that donor funds for HIV and security-related programmes in conflict settings remain limited:

One of the protocols, for instance, for treatment of sexual violence is HIV prophylaxis, and that is not always available, because it's more expensive.... You'd love to apply guidelines and protocols across missions, but you don't have the money to do it. And if we didn't have enough money to do things in Darfur [a lower HIV prevalence region[3]], I would rather convince the donors to provide support for emergency obstetric care than for HIV prophylaxis, because of the very high odds against a rape victim ... getting HIV infected.

(June, 2010)

With limited funds, agencies must engage in a moral calculus wherein forms of care are rationed and unequally distributed across populations and states, and raped women in some regions are left, by virtue of lower national prevalence rates, to assume as individuals the risk of contracting HIV. This is a stark reminder of the extent to which some lives and bodies – mainly those of marginalized women – have not been meaningfully protected by HIV securitization.

The lack of significant new donor contributions for HIV and security programming, especially when new multi-billion dollar commitments were being made elsewhere in the global response, indicates that securitization does not always result in greater resource allocation. Conversely, increased attention and resources can be acquired, as in the case of the Global Fund, without recourse to securitization. Contrary to a widely held expectation of much security studies literature, and of actors leading HIV securitization efforts, positioning something as a security threat is neither sufficient nor necessary to attract significant new resources (for a similar critique, see Rushton, 2010a, 2010b).[4] This does not mean securitizations that fail to produce resource reallocation or broad changes to the social, political and economic landscape are merely 'cheap talk'; securitizing speech acts produce a form of politics in which rule-breaking is tolerated (Buzan et al., 1998), and this rule-breaking often has significant material impact. It does suggest, though, that even securitizations that are successful in producing exceptional threat response may be less effective at achieving other goals relating to resource acquisition. In 'real world' situations, rule-breaking and the circumvention of normal politics are rarely an end in and of themselves; securitizing actors are usually also trying to effect other change, including resource acquisition. The limited ability of HIV securitization in the UNSC to attract significant new funding for the security response to HIV suggests that securitization strategies may not always be an effective means of achieving this type of change.

Organizational change in the UN system

While HIV securitization did not result in immediate or significant changes in HIV spending in the UN, it did produce two organizational changes: the creation of the UNAIDS Office on AIDS, Security and Humanitarian Response (SHR), and a new formalized working relationship between DPKO, UNAIDS and UNFPA.

The SHR office in UNAIDS is meant to coordinate all UN actors implicated in the Resolution 1308 directive. A staff member explained:

> Our role is to provide normative guidance, bring everybody together.... Our job really is to say, "Look, we have a problem here, we have some issue that we need to address; we *know* that you [cosponsoring agencies] are the technical experts ... but we need to have a coordinated response, that people don't go and do whatever, so let's try to work together.... This is how we work, and sometimes it's frustrating, of course, but then that's why we were created, we were created to bring everybody together.
>
> (Ruth, 2009)

This interviewee articulates a core challenge of UNAIDS: to parlay the Secretariat's moral authority and functional responsibility for a coordinated HIV response into technical action on the part of its larger and relatively autonomous co-sponsors.

In the case of the SHR office, this coordinating role would be particularly challenging because it united two programming areas – humanitarian and security programming – that had previously been functionally and conceptually separate in the UN system, and that outside of UNAIDS continued to be treated as distinct categories, each falling under the authority of different bureaucratic actors. Even the SHR unit maintains this structural separation: though overseen by a single Director and holding a comprehensive mandate to address HIV in peacekeeping, uniformed services and humanitarian populations (Joint United Nations Programme on HIV/AIDS (UNAIDS), 2003a, p. 1), the unit is composed of two sections, one responsible for security activities and the other for humanitarian response.

This division between security and humanitarian programming is reflected in most UN agencies, and is exacerbated by the fact that security and humanitarian affairs have also historically been functionally separate from HIV programming. A UNAIDS staff member explained,

> WHO, and UNICEF, UNFPA ... they have their internal HIV departments, and then they have their [humanitarian] emergency departments.... We have been dealing mostly with the HIV departments, so it's been quite a challenge, even within these agencies, to bridge, to get these two departments talking.
>
> (Ruth, 2009)

The implication of the new unit – that HIV required coordinated response from humanitarian, security and HIV actors – thus triggered significant and highly contentious efforts to renegotiate the borders between humanitarian and security programming.

New agreements with implementing agencies were also needed to deliver this new 'security and humanitarian' HIV programming. Because Resolution 1308 focused on peacekeepers, DPKO was necessarily involved. However, since DPKO had neither the mandate nor the technical expertise to provide sexual health programming, UNAIDS also needed a partner agency with the in-house expertise and on-the-ground resources to support this programme delivery. UNFPA had been providing sexual and reproductive health programming to militaries long before Resolution 1308, though not to UN peacekeepers,[5] making it a logical and relatively uncontroversial partner for the 'security' side of the SHR office's activities. It was less clear who should be primarily responsible for implementation on the 'humanitarian' side. Agreements regarding HIV programming in humanitarian emergencies took much longer to develop, and remain contentious (a matter explored later in the chapter).

Assessing the impact of Resolution 1308 in the broader global response to HIV

It is ultimately difficult to assess the extent to which broader shifts in the global response – those outside the remit of security actors or invoking alternate rhetoric and logics, such as human rights, social justice or development – were abetted by the UNSC session and associated securitization efforts. But if we envision a counterfactual situation in which the UNSC did not discuss HIV, and Resolution 1308 was never adopted, there would be little material difference in the global response. The new SHR unit in UNAIDS would likely not have been created, and it is possible that DPKO, UNAIDS and UNFPA would not have entered into a formal partnership to deliver HIV programming to peacekeepers. However, as discussed in the previous chapter, HIV programming for militaries was occurring in and beyond the UN system well before efforts to put HIV on the UNSC agenda. Without Resolution 1308, HIV programming for militaries would still exist, and this programming would reach many of the uniformed services members who might be deployed as peacekeepers. And one of the most significant financial changes in the post-2000 global response, the Global Fund, was not a result of Resolution 1308 or security-specific concerns about HIV, and would have proceeded in the absence of any securitization efforts.[6] Recalling the distinction laid out in the introductory chapter between the securitization of HIV and the broader move to treat HIV as an exceptional emergency, it appears that explicit securitization manoeuvres in the UNSC may have drawn on and reflected this larger sense of urgency, but it is not clear that securitization provided much material 'value added' to these calls for urgent action in the broader global response.

If the immediate material impact of the debate was so limited, if it is difficult to attribute longer-term changes in the global HIV response directly to securitization efforts, and if the significant post-2000 boost in HIV funding was not the result of securitization, why then should we care about Resolution 1308 and the UNSC debates? The answer is that by looking for change in the global response writ large, we are looking in the wrong place. To assess the impact of securitization efforts, we need to examine the policy and programming areas where post-1308 HIV and security work was actually concentrated – peacekeepers and uniformed services – and ask what impact it has had in and through work with the security sector. It is here that we see the subtle but significant effect that HIV and security work has had via the gradual expansion of UN and other global actors' authority into previously domestic spheres, resulting in erosion of sovereignty and bodily autonomy.

To reiterate, neither the limited impact of HIV securitization on the global response writ large, nor the fact that more significant impact has been confined to the security sector, mean that this is a failed securitization. International HIV securitization had already met the CS criteria for successful securitization before Resolution 1308 reached the implementation stage: when the UNSC stated that HIV was a security threat and passed Resolution 1308, this was (1) a securitizing speech act, made by actors in a structural position of authority, invoking existential threat to construct categories of threatened and threatening subjects; that (2) broke the rule that the UNSC deals with military threats, and (3) produced an exceptional threat response not considered necessary, before or since, for any other health issue affecting peacekeepers. The point is precisely that even successful securitizations that set in motion threat response enabling exceptional incursions into bodies and territories may have limited ability to produce other forms of social change.

Boundary work in policy implementation: constructing the 'security response' to HIV

Resolution 1308 established the notional existence of HIV and security as a programme area. But precisely what this programming should entail then needed to be negotiated. This negotiation about the details of Resolution 1308's implementation was largely left to UN bureaucrats. For these actors, 'security programming' implied specific bureaucratic parameters, and where these did not exist they needed to be created to ensure smooth bureaucratic functioning. Ensuing discussions about HIV and security programming were therefore partly logistical: how should programming be coordinated across many semi-autonomous actors, and where does the authority of one agency end and another's begin? These logistical discussions also became a means to renegotiate conceptual categories in the UN bureaucracy, especially the categories of 'security' and 'humanitarian' activity: what do each of these categories mean? Where do their borders overlap, collapse or create gaps that HIV and security programming can fill? These discussions were, essentially, boundary work.

The concept of 'boundary work' has been used to study the rhetorical strategies employed to distinguish 'science' from 'ideology' (Gieryn, 1983), and to show how the boundaries of policy authority are discursively maintained (Scala, 2007). In essence, boundary work is a discursive tactic used by actors to delineate spheres of authority, and to ascribe characteristics to the activities falling within those spheres. This chapter uses the concept to show how UN actors ascribed particular attributes to their own agencies, and to the categories of security and humanitarian activity, in order either to claim these activities as their own, or delegate them to other UN units.

The security–humanitarian divide

Coordinating the security response to HIV required renegotiating the boundaries between security and humanitarian programmes, which historically had been the responsibility of two different sets of actors and agencies. All were territorial, largely unwilling to encourage the encroachment of other agencies onto 'their' turf, and yet, particularly in the case of humanitarian actors, initially reluctant to accept HIV as one of their responsibilities.

One interviewee explained that "for a long time I think [the Security and Humanitarian Response unit] was basically focusing much more on the Security Council resolution, so HIV and security issues, and not so much on humanitarian". She also noted that "from my perspective, the challenge has been getting the humanitarian side and the HIV side to be talking. I think the challenge is less so probably from the security side, because it's quite clear: peacetime, uniformed services" (Ruth, 2009). Another elaborated:

Although there might be some linkages between the humanitarian response and the security, we after several debates and many years of different people coming in and out of the office having the idea that we should have a streamlined agenda, we always ended up keeping them a bit separate ... I mean, there is obviously a role for the security sector or for uniformed services in situations of humanitarian crisis or emergencies, but then in terms of what we do and the global agendas, we keep that a little bit separate because also the architecture of both responses is a bit different.

SH: How is the humanitarian stream different?

RASHMI: [sighs] Uh, because it's a very, I mean, this is clear-cut. This is the scope, these are the sectors, these are the actors.

SH: Security?

RASHMI: Security. So you get down to the job.... Humanitarian is very complicated, because you have UN agencies, but additionally you have mandates for bits and pieces of the humanitarian response, but not for the overall. And then you have discussions between WHO, because HIV is health, and UNHCR because they are [responsible for] refugees and IDPs, so who is going to oversee HIV, the WHO that is responsible for health or the UNHCR that is responsible for refugees and IDPs [internally displaced persons], but then you have people that are in humanitarian situations but are not refugees nor IDPs, and so who is responsible for them, and you have the WFP ...

(Rashmi, 2009)

Boundary work does two things here: first it establishes security programming as activities in the security sector and especially in militaries. Once again, 'security' is immediately understood to refer to the security sector, demonstrating the deeply entrenched meaning of security in the UN system. Boundary work also attributes several characteristics to security activities that distinguish them from humanitarian ones. In particular (and in large part because of the organizational conflation of 'security' with 'militaries'), security becomes "quite clear", "clear-cut" and distinct from "complicated" humanitarian activities where a humanitarian-HIV actor dialogue is "challenging".

Humanitarian actors, also perceiving their frontline activities as highly complex, initially responded to calls for attention to HIV in humanitarian emergencies through boundary work of their own, rejecting the idea that humanitarian programming should encompass HIV prevention and treatment. One interviewee recalled that

all of the mainstream humanitarian actors fought very hard against HIV being part of the repertoire of humanitarian response, because they thought things are hard enough as it is, you know, hard enough to get food into wherever; we can't also start thinking about doing HIV programming.... There was just a general resistance to complicating things.... It's not that people didn't care about HIV, they just didn't think it was a big issue in humanitarian situations.

(June, 2010)

Another observed that:

> Humanitarian, the whole mentality has been ... we're short-term, relief and recovery, and so to bring these [HIV and humanitarian programming] together, again, has been quite challenging, because for a long time people, humanitarians ... they're coming around to it, but for them to address HIV, and the added vulnerability that may be created because of a conflict or a disaster, whatever, it doesn't really come naturally to them because they don't think it's lifesaving, and AIDS ... is a long-term event, you know; you get infected, you have ten years, or five, six years before you're showing AIDS symptoms.

SH: So they're more focused on the short term

RUTH: Yeah, of humanitarian relief ... they say, always, their issue is lifesaving, and AIDS is not lifesaving ... and so for us to get people to come around and say, no, but if you have a crisis in Kenya or something, and people are on ART [anti-retroviral therapy] and you stop their ART, then it *is* potentially lifesaving, or life destroying.

(Ruth, 2009)

One UNAIDS interviewee contended that even now, more than a decade after the move to incorporate HIV programming into humanitarian response, "you still have a lot of people in humanitarian country teams who say, 'Oh, AIDS is not a problem for humanitarian action'" (Keith, 2009).

The UN's humanitarian agencies, then, have historically maintained strong boundaries that keep HIV services provision separate from humanitarian crisis response, and treat both HIV and humanitarian programming as distinct from security programming. What distinguishes these categories is not just the empirical difference between the short time horizon of humanitarian response relative to HIV's long latency period, but also the normative perception that humanitarian programmes are an "emergency response" that is immediately "lifesaving" in a way that HIV prevention and treatment is not. HIV services, rather than being "lifesaving", are understood as further "complicating" humanitarian responses that "are hard enough as it is". The ideas of "lifesaving" and "emergency" operate in the UN to delineate a bureaucratic boundary between humanitarian, HIV, and security spheres. This is an especially stark example of the way that HIV programming in both security and humanitarian sectors has been shaped by UN bureaucratic norms and a preference for "uncomplicated" programme delivery rather than the perspective of those most directly affected by HIV. For people living with HIV who lack treatment access or whose treatment regime is disrupted because of conflict, there is no meaningful boundary between "lifesaving" humanitarian programmes and the provision of HIV treatment: both projects are equally lifesaving.

Crucially, actors engage in boundary work to discursively position "humanitarian response" and programme delivery as an immediately "lifesaving" emergency response, whereas security activities are not. Paradoxically, and contrary to the wide-spread assumption in security studies that it is security, above all else, that confers urgency, emergency and the need for exceptional response, this boundary work makes humanitarian activities – activities that are specifically *not* security activities in the UN lexicon – more urgent, exceptional and "lifesaving" than HIV-related security activities, which are understood as routine, well-structured, clear-cut programming with militaries, addressing non-emergency matters, and operating on a longer time horizon.

DPKO actors were also keen to maintain 'security' as a defined program area focusing on militaries, emphasizing that "our core business will always remain peacekeepers" (Alex, 2010). Maintaining a focus on peacekeepers keeps DPKO's realm of responsibility tightly circumscribed, preventing mission creep (a key concern for the DPKO after the peacekeeping challenges of the 1990s and early 2000s). It also further perpetuates, first, that 'security' refers to militaries, and second, that security activities are distinct from other agencies' complex, overlapping mandates. Security, understood as peacekeeping, is a sphere where DPKO and security actors have primary authority, ensuring "clear-cut" "uncomplicated" division of responsibility.

The consequences of boundary work: security is easy

As a result of boundary work establishing 'security' as specifically 'that pertaining to militaries' and separate from humanitarian programming, the new programming area of HIV and security was initially interpreted in a circumscribed manner: security actors' provision of programming to peacekeepers. This interpretation, and the tendency to conflate security with militaries and the security sector, was facilitated by the formally narrow mandate of Resolution 1308. It was also facilitated by bureaucratic territoriality in the UN system, wherein humanitarian response entails highly contested and overlapping jurisdictions, while security programming is clearly demarcated and agreed to be the responsibility of only a few agencies. However, boundary work equating HIV and security programming with HIV programmes for militaries was soon abetted by the discovery of actors working in this new programming area that security programmes (understood as work with militaries) were not just "clear cut" but also "easy" relative to provision of humanitarian programming.

Several interviewees, for instance, enthused about the merits of the hierarchical structure of militaries for rapidly diffusing information and implementing behavioural interventions. One observed that in working with militaries,

> you've got to get your high-ups believing in it, because if they don't, you're out of luck.... But if you do get them believing in it, it's the easiest group to

work with in the world.... They have a lot of down time, so you can push a lot of information at them, if it's a well-disciplined military and they keep good records and everything; it's much easier programming than it is with any other group.

(June, 2010)

Another interviewee likewise argued that "the military way of doing things is not directly applicable to civil society, but it bloody well works. We're now suggesting you need to do more of these command-centred approaches, get the top leadership, tell these guys what to do" (Keith, 2009).[7]

In addition to the perception that militaries are structurally easy to work with, several interviewees also contended that military leaders tend to have pragmatic and solution-focused attitudes when it comes to HIV and troops' sexual behaviour. Peter Piot, for instance, observed that

> my experience with militaries is that they are actually far less into ... moral types of ideological considerations, about when it comes to sex and all that; they say "OK, well, this is a problem, OK, what can we do? All my men, my boys will need a condom." ... I was pleasantly surprised by the pragmatism of people dealing with security ... I was used to dealing with the public health people, and clergy, and imams, and all that, and oh my god, and then parents' associations, and, phew, you know?

(Piot, 2009)

Security programming, once defined as programming in and for uniformed services, becomes "easy" because of the perceived attributes of militaries. They are hierarchically structured, such that once top leaders are "on board", it is relatively easy to efficiently distribute information. Military leaders are perceived as solution-focused, seeing HIV as primarily a functional, not a moral issue, requiring pragmatic interventions. Militaries are functionally "easier" in terms of the UN division of labour, wherein responsibility for working with militaries is "clear cut" compared to the confusing overlapping jurisdictional authority of humanitarian agencies. Finally, even in the complex environments of peacekeeping missions and other crises, military structures provide access to a clearly defined and easy-to-find population.

Boundary work, then, first established security programming as 'programming with militaries', and second, enabled the discovery that within this circumscribed programming area, 'security is easy'. The result was an enduring categorization norm: HIV securitization failed to dislodge the UN norm that 'security' and 'the security sector' are equivalent categories. The conflation of security with the security *sector* in HIV and security programming solidified the idea that, in the securitized response to HIV, the focal point for intervention is uniformed services and especially militaries – and within that category, especially UN peacekeepers. This in turn reinforced a narrower, national security interpretation of 'HIV is a security threat', with the functional result that HIV was approached not as a broad human security problem, but rather as a threat (mainly emanating from peacekeepers) to the legitimacy and functionality of UN peacekeeping missions.

We can additionally see hints of tension between the logic of securitization, and norms governing humanitarian and community-based HIV responses. Having military leaders "tell these guys what to do" is especially in tension with the norms and ethics of community-based responses emphasizing the importance of individual and community empowerment and autonomy. Further, the belief that 'security is easy' rests on an assumption of homogeneity: militaries are assumed to be male, heterosexual and at risk for sexual transmission of HIV, and it is further assumed that this risk can be mitigated through behavioural interventions to promote condom use. Female peacekeepers, MSM, and people who inject drugs are largely erased from programmes in which condom provision is the programmatic focus. As the perceived easiness of security programming encouraged actors to expand and deepen their HIV and security programmes, these tensions and erasures would be exacerbated, especially when they intersected with gender and human rights concerns.

Pushing the boundaries: contesting the content of HIV and security programming

Initially, the discovery that 'security is easy' referred mainly to the ease with which militaries could be accessed and basic prevention messages disseminated. The discovery that 'security is easy' was soon followed by two related discoveries on the part of those tasked with delivering this programming. First was that basic, in-mission HIV education and condom provision for UN peacekeepers was inadequate. Second was that given the perceived 'easiness' of HIV activities in the security sector, this programming was soon recognized as a convenient means through which other issues, such as human rights and gender, could be brought into military spheres. Finally, highly contentious debates relating to testing and treatment arose as HIV programming in the security sector expanded.

None of these matters were unique to HIV and security programming: the scope of and preferred target audience for prevention education, rules and norms for HIV testing and treatment, and how best to address gender and human rights concerns in HIV programming are routinely debated across the global response. What is notable is what happened to these issues when refracted through the lens of security. Specifically, security-based HIV rhetoric and programming was often in tension with the emancipatory principles of community-based responses to HIV, wherein equity, social justice, human rights and PHA empowerment were central. Even as HIV and security programming gradually began to exceed the scope of Resolution 1308, it remained constrained by the logic of securitization and institutionalized definitions of 'security' in the UN system. That is, the logic of securitization continued to structure the security response to HIV and to determine which interventions this invocation of security authorized and precluded, even as the response expanded.

The widening and deepening of the security response to HIV

The initial focus on in-mission programmes for peacekeepers soon expanded in scope, in part because "there is a turnover of these peacekeeping troops, I think they stay four to six months and that's it. So we said, we need to also look at the troop providers" (Piot, 2009). UN staff tasked with delivering HIV prevention programming further observed that "if you look at 1308 … it's very limited, it's basically training for peacekeepers, it doesn't even say anything about providing counselling or testing" (Maggie, 2010). HIV and security programming therefore began to expand in two ways. First, it grew in temporal scope to encompass programming in pre-and post-deployment periods. Second, it expanded to include a wider range of programming. This 'widening and deepening' of HIV and security programming meant that UN service providers gradually began to reach further into states, accessing not just peacekeepers but members of national militaries who might be deployed as peacekeepers,[8] or who had already returned from deployment to peace missions; they also began to provide a greater range of interventions to regulate the behaviours of these populations, developing HIV education programmes that entailed subtle but deeper encroachments into peacekeepers' bodily autonomy.

An HIV education DVD developed in the mid-2000s illustrates this subtle expansion of programming reach (United Nations Department of Peacekeeping Operations, c. 2004). Intended for peacekeepers in-mission, the DVD begins and ends by emphasizing the UN's zero tolerance policy for sexual abuse and exploitation. Rather than give in to sexual temptation, peacekeepers are instead exhorted to avoid alcohol and pornography, play sports, stay in regular contact with their children and spouse, and remain faithful to that spouse. After presenting this range of sex-prevention strategies, the DVD acknowledges that if peacekeepers do engage in sexual activity, they should use condoms; it also encourages in-mission HIV testing.

The DVD illustrates that HIV prevention for peacekeepers expanded to include not just education about HIV transmission, but also the promotion of particular forms of self-care and self-discipline that comprise a set of practices enacted in, through and upon the body at all times, not just during the actual moments of sexual activity when HIV transmission might occur. The peacekeeper's body is therefore acted upon in a range of subtle but intrusive ways, as behaviours encompassing not just sexual intercourse but sports and leisure activities, consumption of intoxicants and cultivation of particular affective relations with family all become a matter for DPKO and IO intervention. Over time, the security response to HIV then expanded to address a range of bodily practices beyond condom use, and this both required and enabled greater reach of IO actors into national militaries and the intimate bodily practices of peacekeepers. As Elbe (2005) has argued, these efforts to regulate peacekeepers' bodies constitute a form of biopolitical control; as a biopolitical intervention disproportionately targeting African and other global South troops who comprise the majority of peacekeepers, it also has a deeply troubling racial dimension.

The point here is to draw attention to what securitization *does*: the logic of threat construction and response enables deeper IO reach into national militaries and into the bodily practices of peacekeepers than had previously been considered acceptable. In contrast to the contention that these education programmes are merely "examples of good practice … but hardly constitute an exceptional response" (McInnes & Rushton, 2013, p. 14), in fact such prevention programming is predicated precisely upon exceptional intrusions into multiple aspects of peacekeepers' lives, bodies and relationships, justified by virtue of the putative threat they pose. Even if, as members of uniformed services, these peacekeepers were already subject to greater surveillance and control than is usual for civilians, this control had previously been exercised mainly by domestic rather than international actors; and it was predicated on the need to ensure combat-readiness of troops, rather than on the assumption that peacekeepers pose a threat in need of containment. In the security response to HIV, the international extends its reach and influence, and this exceptional threat response is made to seem routine.

Programming also expanded to address a wider range of interactions between peacekeepers and civilians, especially human rights and gender aspects of these interactions. Yet even as they recognized the necessity of addressing these topics, interviewees tasked with implementing HIV programming for peacekeepers perceived that gender and human rights were outside the scope of security programming. "You need an entry point to talk about human rights," one interviewee explained; "I felt that through the issue of HIV/AIDS … we could use that as an entry … when you talk about HIV and AIDS-related discrimination and stigma, then that's where you bring in human rights" (Alex, 2010). He spoke eloquently about protecting the human rights of sex workers, MSM, people who used drugs and other marginalized populations; but despite his deep commitment to human rights education for uniformed services, he still felt "an entry point" was needed for human rights discussions, suggesting that human rights are not, in and of themselves, considered an appropriate topic for uniformed services training.

Similarly, another interviewee contended that

> it can be hard to speak to the military. You want to talk about gender concerns but you can't; but then you talk about how HIV is affecting their military – they care about that – and then you bring in the gender concerns…. You have to find a way to make it relevant to what they think is relevant. Because people dying isn't what makes HIV relevant to everyone, otherwise dysentery would be relevant to everyone, and so would malaria. You've got to put it in their terms.
>
> (Maggie, 2010)

Maggie further suggested that "security is a Trojan horse, what you do is there's certain things you can bring along with it" (2010). The metaphor is apt because while HIV and security actors did indeed use HIV and security programming to smuggle in other messages about human rights and gender, as a Trojan horse, 'security' also carries with it less useful and perhaps harmful baggage, including persistent normative and organizational constraints that structure ideas about what security 'really' means.

To elaborate, human rights and gender were generally seen as issues that needed to be smuggled in to HIV and security programming, carefully positioned to stay relevant to traditional military concerns. This is another powerful indication of deeply entrenched beliefs about the boundaries of security-related activities. The insistence that "people dying" falls outside the ambit of security concerns also echoes Stephen Lewis' remark (cited in Chapter 3) that security and the "life or death" matter of treatment access are separate issues. In sum, security-in-use continues to be understood, even by practitioners expressing human security-like concern for the well-being of people, as *national and international* military security, not human security, and this entrenched belief shapes programming and practices within the security field.

Testing and treatment in the security response to HIV

While the expansion of HIV programming to address gender and human rights required careful positioning, neither this expansion nor efforts to influence a growing range of intimate bodily practices of peacekeepers generated significant controversy among those responsible for security and HIV programming. Instead, testing and treatment – specifically, whether testing should be mandatory or voluntary, and whether treatment should be provided to peacekeepers – became the most contentious issues. It is in these debates where the logic of securitization and the logic of global health are most acutely in tension.

There have been extensive debates in the UN system and in national militaries about whether HIV testing in militaries should be mandatory or voluntary, and whether those who test positive should (1) be allowed to serve in national militaries and (2) be allowed to serve as UN peacekeepers (Elbe, 2009; Keith, 2009; Maggie, 2010). One interviewee, exasperated that these debates have continued, unresolved, from the inception of Resolution 1308 to the present, remarked:

> We need to have an unhysterical discussion about the policy ... you get into a silly discussion, I think, about mandatory testing or not mandatory testing, when really what we probably should be saying is, well look, here's a different category of situation, and a different audience, and you know, if they [militaries] test mandatorily for flat feet, isn't it ridiculous that in these comprehensive health assessments, [they say] "don't test for the disease [HIV]". You can do that confidentially, you can do it with consent, you can do it and make sure that there's decent access to follow-up services for them and their families.... What is not helpful are the people who say ... this is the beginning of a slippery human rights slope.
>
> (Keith, 2009)

Because of continuing tensions between those (mainly in the security sector) supportive of mandatory testing, and others (mainly activists in the broader global response) who are strongly opposed, the DPKO promotes HIV testing in UN peace missions, but has stopped short of implementing mandatory testing. Several troop contributing countries, however, have mandatory testing policies; some also have a policy of not deploying HIV-positive soldiers to UN missions, although the extent to which these policies are followed has been uneven (Bazergan, 2004, p. 5).

Reflecting these tensions, the global response writ large promotes VCT – voluntary counselling and testing – but UN programming for peacekeepers promotes VCCT, voluntary *confidential* counselling and testing. As a DPKO staff explained:

> Here we still use VCCT because we want troop-contributing countries and missions and mission leadership to still understand that that C refers to confidentiality.... In spite of people telling me, "I think we need to align ourselves with common [terminology]" I tell them, "When the time comes, when people understand that confidentiality is taken, is accepted, then we will [use the term VCT] ..."
>
> (Alex, 2010)

Notwithstanding the official DPKO position, there is recognition that for peacekeepers, confidentiality in HIV testing is not guaranteed. A 2004 review acknowledged that "[s]ome military medical officers are expected to inform their commanding officer if a soldier is found to be HIV-positive" and that "there have been cases of military-run medical facilities carrying out precautionary testing on patients prior to basic surgery without the individual's knowledge or consent" (Bazergan, 2004, p. 10). Both the voluntary and confidential aspects of testing, that is, remain more aspirational than actual.

The tension between aspiration and actuality is also reflected in the following description of in-mission HIV testing:

> ALEX: [Peacekeepers] ask, "Will you tell my commander or my medical officer?" "No. We will give you the result, without even your name, but you'll get the result. With a code." And when they walk in [for testing], not one person will walk in, it's one, two, three, he walks in, a little timidity, does it, and he walks out, and people ask him, "What happened?" He'll say, "I got it." "Got what?" "I'm negative." They say, "But you just went in!" "Yeah." "How did they do it?" "They gave it to me." ... He tells his mates, "I got it." "That's all?" "Yeah, that's all." And then the advisor and his team has to tell them, "Look, guys, the chopper is about to leave. And I think we need to close up, and besides we are running out of test kits. So are you going to come?" They say, "Sure, of course we will come." So the demand goes. If they know that you're going to do it with full confidentiality, that's important.
>
> (Alex, 2010)

In the scenario as described, results may formally be confidential, but there is evident peer pressure at work to disclose results, as well as encouragement from field staff to take the test before the mobile team leaves.

There may be merit in as many people as possible being aware of their HIV status, but opportunities for appropriate follow-up are likely to be limited in such already stressful conditions, particularly when mobile testing teams fly in and out of field stations in a single day, leaving behind few staff with HIV expertise. Receiving a positive test result under these circumstances affords little time and privacy to discuss one's options with medical professionals. In militaries barring HIV-positive members, receiving an HIV-positive test can result in job and income loss, exacerbating the stress of an HIV-positive diagnosis. There is then a combined likelihood of being strongly encouraged to seek HIV testing; of one's "mates" naturally being curious about the process and results, possibly compromising confidentiality; of limited follow-up and support; and of potentially severe consequences should one's HIV status become known. This incursion into peacekeepers' bodies remains deeply ethically problematic.

The other option – not offering HIV testing at all if it can only be offered in the suboptimal conditions of many peacekeeping missions – is also ethically problematic, particularly because there is evidence that peacekeepers themselves desire access to VCCT in-mission (Loche & Gurung, 2007). I recount the scenario not to criticize this interviewee's work providing medical care under challenging circumstances, but to reiterate what HIV securitization has made possible: it both normalizes and exacerbates the foreclosure of peacekeepers' bodily autonomy, creating "a different category of situation, and a different audience" (Keith, 2009) in which HIV testing practices that would not be accepted elsewhere in the global response are made to seem necessary and normal. The implication that by virtue of choosing a military career, no matter how constrained that choice might have been, one can then be expected to give up this degree of bodily autonomy and privacy, raises significant ethical questions when applied to HIV testing while deployed. Here, there may be potentially severe repercussions (job loss, stigma, additional psychological stress) yet the intervention may not lead to treatment or other forms of counselling and support at a moment of profound vulnerability. Whose security, exactly, is being defended under these circumstances? This book does not aim to resolve these complex ethical issues, but to illuminate the significant but hidden consequences of HIV securitization.

With respect to HIV treatment, the opposite problem obtains. Here, peacekeepers' bodies more usually remain free of interventions. Post-exposure prophylaxis (PEP) is in principle available[9] for occupational exposure or sexual assault, but treatment is not otherwise routinely provided. While some contend peacekeepers should receive treatment in-mission, especially if they are encouraged to seek testing, others maintain that field medical facilities lack the capacity to provide treatment; that it would become impossible to justify why HIV treatment is offered when treatments for many other illnesses are not; and that because there is no certainty that medicine offered in-mission will be available in home countries, treating HIV in-mission could lead to situations where people start and stop treatment, potentially creating drug resistance (Maggie, 2010). DPKO currently has no guidelines requiring or recommending provision of HIV treatment to peacekeepers in-mission, and few if any in-mission facilities are equipped to provide such care. With the most recent WHO guidelines for HIV treatment now recommending initiation of treatment as soon as possible after diagnosis (World Health Organization (WHO), 2015), this places HIV-related medical care in peace missions and the 'security response' increasingly out of step with best practices in the larger global response.

Human rights are implicated here, too: the right of peacekeepers to access HIV treatment. These rights have been displaced and deferred, as peacekeepers' access to treatment, ability to decline testing, and in some cases, ability to serve if they test HIV-positive, are all restricted. Treatment, already displaced from the category of 'security' in the UNSC sessions through the threat-based logic of securitization and consequent tendency towards defensive threat containment or eradication strategies, now becomes even further functionally set apart from and outside of the security response to HIV. At the bureaucratic and frontline service delivery level, initial securitizing logic is reinforced by perceived functional and logistical impediments to treatment; that is, with the exception of PEP, HIV treatment is perceived as something that cannot feasibly be provided to peace-keepers in-mission. Once again, securitization creates "a different category of situation" where failing to provide treatment is made to seem acceptable, normal, and unavoidable.[10]

Approaches to HIV testing and treatment in the security response to HIV highlight ongoing tensions between the logics of securitization and health, and the different relations with peacekeepers' bodies these logics entail. In the broader global response, principles of equity, social justice and PHA empower-ment have been central. But in the security response to HIV, the operational requirements of peacekeeping operations and military preparedness have trumped medical best practice standards for treatment and social justice demands for equity and universal treatment access. Through this same securitizing logic, while treatment is placed outside the security response, testing and other preven-tion efforts become easier. Here, using hierarchical structures to enforce behavi-oural interventions and promote HIV testing has meant that many of the challenges inherent in community-based HIV work are stripped away. The need for consent, participatory approaches and PHA leadership in all aspects of pro-gramming, foundational to community responses, is largely absent in HIV and security programming. Precisely the coercive, stigmatizing and intrusive forms of biopolitical control hypothesized by Elbe (2009) have eventuated in the response to HIV in peacekeeping and conflict settings.

Conclusion: Silence, exclusion and the inversion of ends and means

The policy implementation stage of HIV securitization was characterized by ongoing tensions and meaning-making contests in the UN bureaucracy over what HIV and security programming ought to entail, and which bureaucratic actors should be responsible. These contests were managed in large part through boundary work, which first served to cordon off HIV and security programming, limiting it to the security sector. This has had the effect of making Resolution 1308, as a securitized response to HIV, seem narrow, limited, and perhaps trivial in its impact, especially since the greatest successes in the larger global response (those relating to increased funding and ARV access) were not achieved via securitization.

But within the carefully delineated sphere comprising the 'security response to HIV', programming then expanded in ways that supported growing reach of the international into the bodies and behaviours of peacekeepers, with potentially severe consequences. Ideas about 'security' also worked to enable the suppression of rights considerations (especially with respect to peacekeeper testing and treatment), thereby becoming a way to deny or limit treatment access rather than expand it. In this manner, the initial aim of HIV securitization – improving HIV programming and treatment access in the global response – was transformed from an end goal into the means to a different end: securing some bodies and states from the threat posed by other bodies and states. There was a reversal of ends and means in which the logic of securitization, not the activist logic of health and social justice (especially the imperative for universal treatment access), ultimately triumphed.

This analysis reveals a troubling relationship between securitization and sovereignty, suggesting that securitization simultaneously worked to defend the sovereignty of some bodies and states while authorizing transgression of and into others. When Resolution 1308 was passed, Holbrooke insisted that it "in no way infringes on the sovereignty or authority of countries" (Holbrooke in United Nations Security Council, 2000). This claim was only partially correct. The sovereignty of some countries, mainly global North states that are not significant troop contributors or receivers, did remain largely unaffected by Resolution 1308. HIV and security programming, though, especially as it expanded over time, constituted a deeper incursion of international actors into national militaries and the lives of some uniformed services members, especially those in the global South states that are the largest troop contributors. This programming, initially tightly circumscribed, gradually expanded to include pre- and post-deployment periods, gender and human rights education, HIV testing, and a range of strategies to influence peacekeepers' bodily practices.

However, the organizational conflation of security with the security sector, and boundary work to maintain the division between security and humanitarian programming, continued to curtail and constrain the scope and nature of the security response to HIV, resulting in continued silences and exclusions. Because of the enduring categorization norm that 'security' refers to the security sector, many other aspects of the global HIV pandemic (for example the Eastern European and Southeast Asian pandemics largely driven by drug use and sex work) were erased or overlooked in the security response. HIV securitization in the UN, that is, did not extend to these locations, populations or modes of transmission, which comprised a significant (though still small relative to sub-Saharan Africa) component of the global pandemic. By equating HIV securitization with HIV prevention programming in UN peace missions, larger structural and redistributive interventions were placed outside of the security response. Securitization facilitated more robust HIV prevention programming and testing in peacekeeping missions, but did not catalyse action beyond the security sector or outside of the narrow logic of threat response.

Africa too became less visible and overtly acknowledged as HIV and security programming was implemented. The urgency of the African pandemic, which had ostensibly been the impetus for initial efforts to securitize HIV, was nowhere evident in the security response rolled out after Resolution 1308. At the programme implementation stage, Africa was far less visible, and its pandemic remained largely unaddressed by the security response to HIV. While African states continued to host the majority of peacekeeping missions in the years following Resolution 1308, and to contribute the bulk of troops to those missions, they were the implicit rather than the explicit focus of HIV and security programming; and in any event these peacekeepers remained a miniscule minority of the global population living with and affected by HIV. African women, in particular, remained almost entirely absent from HIV and security work except where they were the sexual partners of uniformed services; high-prevalence southern African states that were neither troop contributors nor hosts of peacekeeping missions were likewise excluded from the peacekeeping-focused security response to HIV. While these other regions and populations were and continue to be addressed through other, non-security-based programming, the central point here is that these were left out of the security response to HIV, even though they were invoked in the initial securitizing moves that constructed HIV as a security threat, and even though, empirically, these regions and populations, not peacekeepers, were the ones most deeply affected by HIV. Africa, having served its rhetorical purpose in threat construction, was disappeared in threat response.

Recalling the framework presented in Chapter 2, suggesting that the relationship between securitization and desecuritization be understood as a Möbius strip in which one state bleeds into the other, we can see that HIV securitization entailed the continuity of some elements of normal politics, as it built upon prior, existing programmes in and with uniformed services. It also entailed the continuity of exceptionalism as programming was implemented through the bureaucratic structures of the UN system. HIV securitization produced exceptional if localized threat response: UN peace missions now include HIV advisors, and robust education and behavioural intervention programming unique to HIV. HIV testing and the robustness with which this testing is promoted is also, because of HIV-related stigma and the potentially severe consequences of testing positive, more intrusive than testing for other common health conditions and diseases, making this too an exceptional aspect of the security response to HIV.

Yet the exceptionality of HIV securitization has become somewhat elided, in part because the circumstances of peace missions are thought to make some forms of HIV programming, such as provision of treatment, impossible; and others, such as potentially non-confidential testing, merely a function of how militaries work. In this manner, the exceptional becomes normalized and unremarkable. Additionally, components of this exceptional programming response are operationalized through the bureaucratic structures of UN agencies like UNFPA, which appear to operate in the realm of normal politics, and this has the effect of folding exceptional threat response into bureaucratic routine. At both ends of the securitization process, the normal and the exceptional are co-mingled, and the exceptional is made to seem both routine and detached from the securitizing speech act in which it originated.

In sum, when urgency met bureaucracy, the resulting security response to HIV had significant and in many respects problematic impact within UN peace missions, while having little impact on the broader global response or the populations most affected by HIV. Over the following decade, this security response to HIV would continue to expand, quietly and in the seemingly unexceptional structures and practices of routine UN programming, until it came to constitute the 'everyday exceptionalism' explored in the following chapter.

Notes

1 UNAIDS reported HIV allocations rose from US$316 million in 1999 to US$1.1 billion in 2000, US$1.3 billion in 2001 and US$1.9 billion in 2002 (UNAIDS Programme Coordinating Board, 2002). A subsequent independent evaluation shows an increase in global HIV spending from just under US$1,000 million in 1999 to almost US$2,000 million in 2001, US$3,000 million in 2002, over US$4,000 million in 2003, US$6,000 million in 2004 and just over US$8,000 million in projected spending in 2005 (ITAD and HLSP, 2008). A 2008 UNAIDS report indicates spending rose to US$10 billion in 2007 (Joint United Nations Programme on HIV/AIDS (UNAIDS), 2008). The trend of significant spending increases post-2000 is consistent across sources.

2 There was a shift from each cosponsoring agency making separate requests to donors for HIV-related programming, to the development of a UNAIDS Unified Budget and Workplan (UBW) which integrated all HIV activities and associated budgets. This allowed donors to make a single payment to the UBW (overseen by UNAIDS) rather than smaller piecemeal commitments across the UN system. Consequently, funds that would previously have been reported within cosponsoring agencies' budgets are now reported as UNAIDS funds.

3 HIV prevalence in Sudan was approximately 1.4% in 2008 (Joint United Nations Programme on HIV/AIDS (UNAIDS), 2008).

4 Harman (2010) has further argued that the World Bank (acting almost entirely outside the 'security response' to HIV, and with very little visibility) is responsible for catalysing some of the most significant changes in the HIV response, which have transformed IO-national government-civil society relations in much of sub-Saharan Africa.

5 UNFPA works with militaries to reach cohorts of young people with family planning information. A senior staff member of UNFPA recalled that prior to Resolution 1308, "at one point somebody in UNFPA was saying, 'we have a division of labour with UNAIDS, and nobody has said anything about uniformed services yet, so should we be doing this work [HIV education in militaries]?' And we said ... in that division of labour, UNFPA is responsible for young people.... Well, these are young people, right? So we kind of came at it from that angle" (June, 2010). The

anecdote is illustrative of the ways that actors dealing with the relatively new issue area of HIV interpreted new work through existing organizational divisions of labour.

6 It is possible that the Global Fund would not have received as much money from donor states had they not made public commitments in and around the time of the UNSC sessions. But this does not indicate the success of securitization *qua* securitization; it merely affirms that it is easier to hold an actor accountable for a commitment made in public.

7 These observations may however overstate the efficacy of command structures. A programme review in Sierra Leone (UNAMSIL) found significant inconsistencies in programme quality (Bazergan, 2002), underscoring disparities between UN headquarters' staff perception of policy implementation, and the 'on the ground' view from peacekeeping missions.

8 Pre-deployment training is nominally the responsibility of troop contributors, but DPKO provides support including material and personnel who deliver pre-deployment training sessions (Joint United Nations Programme on HIV/AIDS (UNAIDS), 2005).

9 In peacekeeping missions the full 28-day cycle is provided, in contrast to other UN sites where a three-day course is started and staff are then repatriated. However, the extent to which PEP is actually available may vary by mission (Bazergan, 2002).

10 This finding is at odds with the warning that treating HIV as a security problem may result in uniformed services gaining preferential access to ARVs. While there is some evidence (Elbe 2006, p. 129) that at the national level, higher-ranking uniformed services members in some states have been given preferential access to scarce essential medicines (which may be due as much or more to their socioeconomic status, not simply the fact of their military service), those deployed as peacekeepers appear to have limited to no access to treatment. Here, securitization logic produces entirely the opposite result, using the exigencies of conflict to justify restricted treatment access for uniformed services.

References

Alex (2010, 12 April). (Personal interview with author.)

Bazergan, Roxanne. (2002). HIV/AIDS & peacekeeping: a field study of the policies of the United Nations Mission in Sierra Leone. London: The International Policy Institute, King's College London.

Bazergan, Roxanne. (2004). HIV/AIDS: Policies and programs for Blue Helmets. *Institute for Security Studies Paper 96*. Pretoria: Institute for Security Studies.

Buzan, Barry, Wæver, Ole, & de Wilde, Jaap. (1998). *Security: A New Framework for Analysis*. Boulder, CO: Lynne Rienner.

Elbe, Stefan. (2005). AIDS, security, biopolitics. *International Relations*, *19*(4), 403–419.

Elbe, Stefan. (2009). *Virus Alert: Security, Governmentality, and the AIDS Pandemic*. New York: Columbia University Press.

Gieryn, Thomas F. (1983). Boundary-work and the demarcation of science from non-science: strains and interests in professional ideologies of scientists. *American Sociological Review*, *48*(6), 781–795.

Gray, Dylan Mohan (Writer). (2012). *Fire in the blood*. In Dylan Mohan Gray (Producer). Ireland: Dartmouth Films & Films Transit.

Harman, Sophie. (2010). *The World Bank and HIV/AIDS: Setting a Global Agenda*. New York: Routledge.

ITAD and HLSP. (2008). The second independent evaluation of UNAIDS, 2002–2008 inception report. UK: ITAD and HLSP for UNAIDS.

Joint United Nations Programme on HIV/AIDS (UNAIDS). (2003a). On the Front Line: A Review of Policies and Programmes to Address HIV/AIDS Among Peacekeepers and Uniformed Services (1st ed.). Copenhagen: UNAIDS Office on AIDS, Security and Humanitarian Response, UN Nordic Office.

Joint United Nations Programme on HIV/AIDS (UNAIDS). (2003b). UNAIDS Office on AIDS, security and humanitarian response annual update 2003. Copenhagen: UNAIDS Office on AIDS, Security and Humanitarian Response.

Joint United Nations Programme on HIV/AIDS (UNAIDS). (2004). UNAIDS Office on AIDS, security and humanitarian response 3rd quarterly report 2004. Copenhagen: UNAIDS Office on AIDS, Security and Humanitarian Response.

Joint United Nations Programme on HIV/AIDS (UNAIDS). (2005). *On The Front Line: A Review of Policies and Programmes to Address AIDS Among Peacekeepers and Uniformed Services* (5th ed.). New York: UNAIDS, SHR New York Office.

Joint United Nations Programme on HIV/AIDS (UNAIDS). (2008). 2008 Report on the global AIDS epidemic. Geneva: Joint United Nations Programme on HIV/AIDS (UNAIDS).

June (2010, 23 April). (Personal interview with author.)

Kapstein, Ethan B. & Busby, Joshua W. (2013). *AIDS Drugs for All: Social Movements and Market Transformations*. Cambridge, UK: Cambridge University Press.

Keith (2009, 27 October; 18 November). (Personal interview with author).

Lewis, Stephen (2011, 17 January). (Personal interview with author).

Loche, Elisabeth & Gurung, Dr. Megh. (2007). *HIV/AIDS Knowledge, Attitude and Practice Survey: UN Uniformed Peacekeepers in Haiti*. New York: United Nations Department of Peacekeeping Operations (DPKO) Peacekeeping Best Practices Section.

Maggie (2010, 4 June). (Personal interview with author.)

McInnes, Colin & Rushton, Simon. (2010). HIV, AIDS and security: where are we now? *International Affairs, 86*(1), 225–245.

McInnes, Colin & Rushton, Simon. (2013). HIV/AIDS and securitization theory. *European Journal of International Relations, 19*(1), 115–138.

Patrick (2009, 14 December). (Personal interview with author).

Piot, Peter (2009, 23 October). (Personal interview with author).

Rashmi (2009, 28 October). (Personal interview with author).

Rushton, Simon. (2010a). AIDS and international security in the United Nations system. *Health Policy and Planning, 25*, 495–504.

Rushton, Simon. (2010b). Framing AIDS: securitization, development-ization, rights-ization. *Global Health Governance, 4*(2), 1–17.

Ruth (2009, 9 November). (Personal interview with author).

Scala, Francesca. (2007). Scientists, government and "boundary work": the case of reproductive technologies and genetic engineering in Canada. In Michael Orsini & Miriam Smith (Eds.), *Critical Policy Studies* (pp. 211–231). Vancouver: UBC Press.

Smith, Raymond A. & Siplon, Patricia D. (2006). *Drugs Into Bodies: Global AIDS Treatment Activism*. Westport, CT: Praeger.

The Global Fund to Fight AIDS, Tuberculosis and Malaria. (2002). Press release 7 July 2002: First Global Fund grants make possible six-fold increase in ARV treatment in Africa. Retrieved 12 February 2012 from www.theglobalfund.org/en/mediacenter/pressreleases/2002-07-07_First_Global_Fund_Grants_Make_Possible_Six-Fold_Increase_in_ARV_Treatment_in_Africa/.

The Global Fund to Fight AIDS, Tuberculosis and Malaria. (2012). About the Global Fund: our history. Retrieved 12 February 2012 from www.theglobalfund.org/en/about/secretariat/history/.

UNAIDS Programme Coordinating Board. (2002). Five-year evaluation of UNAIDS. Geneva: UNAIDS Programme Coordinating Board.

United Nations Department of Peacekeeping Operations. (*c.*2004). *Hidden Risk: HIV and Peacekeeping* [DVD].

United Nations Security Council. (2000). Transcript: Agenda: The responsibility of the Security Council in the maintenance of international peace and security: HIV/AIDS and international peacekeeping operations (Security Council 55th year, 4172nd meeting, Monday 17 July 2000 S/PV.4172).

World Health Organization (WHO). (2015). Treat all people living with HIV, offer antiretrovirals as additional prevention choice for people at "substantial" risk. Retrieved 18 January 2016 from www.who.int/mediacentre/news/releases/2015/hiv-treat-all-recommendation/en/.

6 Through the looking glass
The production of HIV and security knowledge

The previous chapter demonstrated that HIV and security programming was quietly expanded during the programme implementation stage that followed Resolution 1308. This work was for the most part submerged, occurring in and through the bureaucratic structures of the UN system. Over the next decade, international politics and the UNSC agenda were dominated by crises and securitizations other than HIV, which seemed, following the high-water mark of global treatment access activism and funding announcements in the early 2000s, to somewhat recede as an international political concern. When I visited Geneva in October 2009, though, several UN staff informed me with much excitement that planning was underway for another HIV-focused UNSC session, coinciding with the tenth anniversary of Resolution 1308, which would reaffirm and expand HIV and security work. They expected a high-profile debate, the centerpiece of which would be the then just-released AIDS, Security and Conflict Initiative (ASCI) report (de Waal et al., 2010), authored by several prominent HIV and security analysts. But January 2010 came and went with no tenth-anniversary session ... and then so did January 2011. Eventually, in June 2011, the UNSC held a brief session to adopt Resolution 1983, which reaffirms the need to address HIV, including through strategies to address sexual violence, in peacekeeping, conflict and post-conflict peacebuilding. Although placing HIV and security in a broader context of conflict and post-conflict peacebuilding, Resolution 1983's action items were simply an affirmation of current work. Unlike the sessions in 2000, this meeting and resolution received no media attention, and it was hardly the high-profile debate and call for action that my interviewees had anticipated.

Resolution 1983's apparent lack of substance and failure to garner significant media or member state attention may suggest that HIV's 'security moment' has passed, with UNSC securitization efforts having failed to achieve any lasting change in the global response (McInnes & Rushton, 2013; Rushton, 2010). Yet Resolution 1983 and surrounding discourse, which relied heavily on the ASCI report, at once reconceptualized the relationship between HIV, security and peacekeeping in a manner that refuted most of the foundational assumptions of Resolution 1308, *and* still insisted that HIV is a security threat. In this sense Resolution 1983 and the ASCI report demonstrate not that HIV is desecuritized, but rather that 'HIV is a security threat' is a remarkably persistent idea, the meaning and content of which has also evolved significantly. The continued efforts of some actors to position HIV as a security threat, now using 'though the looking glass' arguments contradictory to those employed ten years earlier to justify the same positioning, suggests that securitizing actors learn over time. Further, when we examine how and from whom securitizing actors learned, we find evidence that HIV securitization has been an iterative strategic practice produced through interactions between security analysts and practitioners.

To demonstrate that the evolution of HIV securitization has entailed an iterative process of actor learning, and a mutually constitutive relationship between security theory and practice, this chapter first traces how the meaning of 'HIV is a security threat' in Resolution 1983 and the ASCI report differs from the meaning of the same statement in Resolution 1308 and related HIV securitization efforts in 2000. It argues that the expansive HIV and security programming endorsed by the ASCI report has come to constitute a form of everyday exceptionalism in which incursions into bodies and territories are accomplished via the desecuritized realm of bureaucratic politics, where the HIV-security nexus has become the domain of an epistemic community of HIV and security experts. Second, drawing on May's (1992) typology of policy learning, the chapter shows that these HIV and security experts then learned from each other, producing HIV and security as a field of expert knowledge and at the same time transforming the meaning of 'HIV is a security threat'. The chapter concludes by discussing the implications of this analysis, chiefly that actor-analyst interactions render securitization theory inherently political, in ways that deeply implicate the theory in the 'real world' securitizations that it studies.

Redefining HIV and security: the ASCI report and Resolution 1983

The ASCI report

Following the UNSC debates, there was increasing interest in HIV and security, particularly in applied and policy-relevant research, among academics and policy makers in the security sector. In response to this interest, the AIDS, Security and Conflict Initiative (ASCI) was convened in 2005. The initiative commissioned research projects including on military and uniformed services; humanitarian crisis and post-conflict transitions; fragile states; gender; and data interpretation (de Waal et al., 2010, p. 16), which fed into a summary document providing overarching findings and policy recommendations. This final report, *HIV/AIDS, Security and Conflict: New Realities, New Responses*, was released in late 2009 and was expected to be the core document informing the planned tenth-anniversary UNSC session. It was also anticipated that the report's guidelines would catalyse further HIV and security programming in and beyond the UN.

The report appropriates the language of securitization, but presents HIV securitization as an unproblematic, positive move, with no acknowledgement that much securitization theory holds a general preference for desecuritization, or that securitization is typically conceived in academic literature as a strategy to circumvent normal politics and to justify rule-breaking and exceptional practices. The report findings also challenge several of the foundational assumptions that drove HIV securitization in 2000, including that peacekeepers are vectors for HIV transmission, that HIV risk is most acute during periods of war and armed conflict, and that high HIV prevalence rates pose a direct threat to state stability. The report suggests that

> [b]y redefining the contours and fault lines of what has hitherto been a largely political debate influenced by speculation and foreign policy concerns as much as by evidence, ASCI identifies new opportunities and strategies for HIV/AIDS prevention and response within uniformed services and fragile states and during humanitarian crises and post conflict transitions.
>
> (de Waal et al., 2010, p. 66)

This strategic positioning of the report presents the claims that initially drove international HIV securitization as largely disproven, distancing itself – and by implication the report authors – from these claims. It does so by invoking the rhetoric of evidence, presenting ASCI report findings as separate from the earlier, "largely political debate" that produced these erroneous assertions. Whereas HIV and security debates in 2000 were "speculative" and "political", the discussions engendered by this report are now evidence-based and, presumably, outside of politics. Scientific inquiry here performs many of the same functions as securitization, namely lifting an issue out of politics and demarcating it as an area of expert authority, beyond political critique and debate. A teleological narrative of progress positions HIV and security researchers and practitioners as experts, and positions HIV and security policy as a site of specific technical, not political, expertise. The locus of power and authority is thereby transferred from political leaders (in, for example, the UNSC), to the technical, bureaucratic and academic experts who have produced and hold mastery over this new evidence-based policy area. This entrenches HIV and security experts as authorities, outside of politics, whose power and expertise flows objectively and unproblematically from evidence, not the "speculation" and "foreign policy concerns" of political actors.

The report recommends expanded HIV and security programming, which in turn further entrenches expert authority in the bureaucratic and military organizational structures through which programming is implemented. Recommendations include expansion of programming to post-conflict and fragile states; expansion to other uniformed services; use of uniformed services' command structure to implement interventions; use of uniformed services as HIV educators; and alignment of strategies to address HIV with strategies to prevent and address sexual violence. As discussed in the previous chapter, much of this work was already being done 'under the radar' by UN staff tasked with delivering HIV and security programming, so the report effectively constitutes, using an appeal to evidence-based policy, a rationale for continuing in a more overt and systematic manner the programming that had already been quietly, incrementally implemented over the previous ten years.

In addition to the ASCI report mainly reiterating support for existing practices rather than proposing genuinely new work, the evidence presented in the report is not novel. A 2005 report produced by the Council on Foreign Relations (Garrett, 2005, pp. 9–10) reached essentially the same conclusions, and by 2010 the foundational assertions of Resolution 1308 and initial HIV securitization had already been challenged by many academics (T. Barnett & Prins, 2006; McInnes, 2006; Whiteside, de Waal & Gebre-Tensae, 2006), including some (de Waal, 2006; Elbe, 2006) whose initial work provisionally accepted early assertions about causal links between HIV, conflict and security (de Waal, 2003; Elbe, 2003).

McInnes and Rushton (2013, p. 17) suggest that the ASCI report's finding that "a number of earlier, more alarmist relationships that were assumed to exist between national-level state security and HIV and AIDS are not borne out by the evidence" (de Waal et al., 2010, p. 12) indicates the desecuritization of HIV. Yet the report uses evidence precisely to support a renewed and refined understanding of how and why HIV *is* a security threat, even using the language of securitization to promote this positioning. Indeed, the very next sentence of the report states that "ASCI also identifies very specific threats posed by HIV ... [and] highlights under-examined HIV risks in humanitarian emergencies and post-conflict transition and in situations of fragility" (de Waal et al., 2010, p. 12). The ASCI report does not appear to support HIV desecuritization, nor was this how the report was received by key stakeholders, including UNAIDS staff responsible for supporting delivery of HIV and security programming, who regarded ASCI findings as a strong statement in support of their work in the 'security response' to HIV, and the continued treatment of HIV as a security threat.

UN staff working on HIV and security programming anticipated that ASCI recommendations would provide the framework for a new UNSC resolution validating their current programming and facilitating its expansion. One analyst explained that

> now the advocacy is not that we have to work with these [uniformed services] populations, I think that message is quite well sunk in. Now the message is, we need to sustain our programmes, and we really need to scale up and strengthen services, and build capacity.... The Security Council report hopefully will give us good recommendations ... on how to take the area forward.
>
> (Cindy, 2010)

In particular, she identified the need for better linkages between HIV and gender programmes in peacekeeping, and hoped that the ASCI report and UNSC session would provide a high-level directive to strengthen and expand this work in a more structured manner. Indeed, Resolution 1983, by explicitly calling for the linkage of HIV-related programming to broader efforts to address sexual violence and the needs of women and girls in peacekeeping operations, provided precisely this directive. A UNAIDS manager elaborated:

> This [ASCI report] says that ... the evidence doesn't support what the Resolution [1308] was based on. But now is not the time to drop the ball, on the contrary. What we're trying to do is reframe this resolution and say ... we were looking in the wrong places.... We don't have a sufficient evidence base to make these calculations about the effects of HIV and AIDS on state fragility because we don't know how to measure state fragility. We don't have it to even talk about national and international security.... We like this report very much ... saying look, you've got to be more nuanced about this. You've missed opportunities. What the evidence does show is that the post-conflict transition period is the period that you need to be paying greater attention to.... There's a captive audience around the DDR [disarmament, demobilization and reintegration] programmes, we haven't done enough work on that.... We dived into the water, went straight to conflict, and came up with all the wrong ideas.... So I think what we're trying to do in the report to the Security Council this time is say, OK, you weren't idiots, it wasn't the wrong thing to do, you did a very good thing, and in fact there's tremendous benefits and spin-offs from having that Security Council resolution, not just for peacekeepers, which it was designed to address, but for the AIDS response in general. So that was great. But let's be a bit more nuanced in what we do. Let's now look at what the evidence is showing, and try to address it.
>
> (Keith, 2009)

Later in the same interview, he returned to the fact that ASCI report findings do not support the foundational assertions of Resolution 1308:

> One of the things that the jury is still out on a little bit, but I think ASCI was really good at highlighting, was the common myth upon which the first Security Council resolution was based, around peacekeepers having higher prevalence than the host communities. I mean even if it was true, it's such a narrow vision that it's not helpful in the work towards universal access.... What we're saying is that there's a mess of opportunity here that we haven't harnessed, which was perhaps the root of the resolution, but which was not harnessed.
>
> (Keith, 2009)

This interviewee recognizes that several foundational assumptions of international HIV securitization in 2000, including that there is a demonstrable causal link between HIV incidence, state fragility and national security, and that peacekeepers are especially likely to contract and transmit HIV, are not supported by evidence. In the absence of this causal link, Resolution 1308's rationale for HIV securitization evaporates, since there is no longer evidence to suggest that HIV poses an existential threat to states or peacekeepers. Yet there is clear desire to nevertheless keep using security rhetoric to promote attention to HIV, and to use the mechanism of UNSC resolutions to secure support for programme expansion with a view to harnessing "missed opportunities". Following from the perception that invoking security continues to have strategic utility, is the desire to use the security response to HIV to promote universal treatment access and to improve "the AIDS response in general". This indicates that actors tasked with executing the security response to HIV continue to regard securitization as a promising strategy to address HIV, even if the invocation of security now requires significant, deliberate revisions to the meaning of 'HIV is a security threat' because "the evidence doesn't support what the Resolution [1308] was based on". They especially (and correctly) see treatment access as a persistent unmet need – although this aspect of the global HIV response has not been successfully securitized or folded into Resolution 1983.

Resolution 1983

Resolution 1983 is clearly shaped by the ASCI report language and findings, stating that HIV may be a greater threat in post-conflict situations, and framing peacekeepers as educators. Resolution 1983 begins with an acknowledgment of Resolution 1308, and then lists a range of other "relevant resolutions" including Resolution 1325 (a precedent-setting resolution calling for gender mainstreaming in peacekeeping and peacebuilding activities) and others addressing sexual violence, exploitation and gender and/in conflict, peace operations and post-conflict peacebuilding, including security sector reform (SSR) and disarmament, demobilization and reintegration (DDR). Notably, these other resolutions, in many respects more expansive in scope than Resolution 1308, did not mention HIV or Resolution 1308. Resolution 1983 then elaborates upon the connection between gender, conflict and sexual violence, the impact of HIV on peacekeeping personnel, and the relationship between conflict, post-conflict, gender-based violence, and HIV transmission. It concludes by encouraging the continuation and full implementation of existing policies and programmes.

By describing HIV and security programming in this expansive manner, it knits together two strands of recurring UNSC discussions that had heretofore been separate: those relating to gender and sexual violence, and those relating to HIV. Crucially, however, it does so by affirming the need to continue and expand existing HIV-related programmes. That is, rather than requesting urgent new rule-breaking projects, Resolution 1983 affirms programming that, thirteen years after Resolution 1308, is now entrenched in UNAIDS and its partner agencies' bureaucracies. This is not to say that Resolution 1983 was ineffective: as interviewees had hoped, it constitutes formal (if *ex post facto*) UNSC recognition that initially narrowly-conceived HIV and security work with peacekeepers is and should continue to be connected to much broader policy and programming dealing with gender, sexual violence and post-conflict peacebuilding. Having formal endorsement of this wider understanding of how and to whom HIV is a security threat undoubtedly provides additional leverage for staff working on HIV and security programming, as it confers legitimacy on activities already underway.

HIV has not been desecuritized, but rather the idea 'HIV is a security threat', as well as subsequent rule-breaking and exceptional programming initiated by Resolution 1308 and endorsed by Resolution 1983, have become so accepted and common-place that they have settled into the realm of routine, bureaucratic procedures. The *securitized response* to HIV is now being delivered through the organizational structures and practices of normal politics. This has been accomplished, furthermore, by advancing a quite different understanding of how, why and to whom HIV is a threat than was articulated in Resolution 1308.

Through the looking glass: HIV and security in 2000 and 2011

When we compare discussions of how, why and to whom HIV is a security threat in the ASCI report, the 2011 Security Council session and Resolution 1983 to the initial articulations of 'HIV is a security threat' in 2000, significant differences emerge (see Table 6.1). Some aspects of the initial construction have been erased entirely, others magnified, and still others inverted so that claims are now being made that contradict assertions made in 2000. At the same time that HIV and security discourse has passed 'through the looking glass' to encompass claims incompatible with those upon which the initial UNSC discussions were based, there are some enduring continuities, which produce continued discursive and programmatic constraints.

Africa's absence

One of the most striking aspects of the discussion of HIV in 2000 and 2011 is the shifting position of Africa, which is not mentioned at all in Resolution 1983. Resolution 1983 specifies that HIV can be exacerbated in conflict and post-conflict situations, and that women and girls are especially affected by HIV (United Nations Security Council, 7 June 2011, paras. 10 & 11) – two aspects of the HIV – security nexus that went unmentioned in 2000. No mention, however, is made of the fact that sub-Saharan Africa is the region with the highest HIV prevalence rates in the world, nor that the feminization of HIV is particularly acute in that region. Africa is likewise not an explicit focal point of the ASCI report, though eight of the commissioned research reports have an empirical African focus, and other reports make reference to particular African states. Furthermore, while the geographic focus of HIV and security discourse has shifted from Africa to areas of conflict and post-conflict, this elides the reality that many of those areas are African. In 2011, then, we see further discursive erasure of Africa in HIV and security discourse in the UNSC, even as the material impact of HIV continued to be greatest on that continent, and even as, in practical terms,

Table 6.1 HIV and security in 2000 and 2011

		HIV and security in 2000: Resolution 1308	HIV and security in 2011: Resolution 1983 and the ASCI report
Threat construction	**Referent object: *to whom* is HIV a threat?**	States and state stability	Women and girls (via sexual violence); UN peacekeeping missions personnel
	***How* is HIV a threat? *Where does* the threat originate?**	High rates of HIV will lead to state collapse; may impede effectiveness of peacekeeping operations. HIV is spread by peacekeepers	Sexual violence in conflict and post-conflict may spread HIV and inhibit post-conflict peacebuilding; may impede effectiveness of peacekeeping operations. HIV is spread through sexual violence
Programming implications	**Peacekeepers' roles**	Peacekeepers are vectors/threats	Peacekeepers are educators and service providers
	Target populations	UN peacekeeping personnel	Uniformed services (including military, police, customs agents and other domestic uniformed services); civilians (especially women and girls) in conflict and post-conflict situations
	Gendered analysis	No mention of gender (but programming largely assumes male peacekeepers)	Significant focus on gender (the particular vulnerability of women and girls) and sex and gender-based violence
	Temporal scope	Duration of peacekeeping operations (de facto expansion to pre-deployment training)	Peacekeeping operations and post-conflict peacebuilding, including security sector reform (SSR) and disarmament, demobilization and reintegration (DDR)
	Geographic scope	Peacekeeping operations, with specific mention of sub-Saharan Africa	Peacekeeping operations and areas of conflict and post-conflict, with no mention of Africa
	Scope of UN-led programming	HIV prevention education for peacekeepers	HIV awareness and outreach to civilians in peacekeeping zones; prevention, testing; zero-tolerance of sexual exploitation and abuse; use of "command-centred approach"; treatment "as appropriate" (but in practice, limited)

HIV and security programming continued to at once disproportionately implicate African troop-contributing and receiving states, while failing to reach more deeply affected populations outside these states.

As in 2000, African representatives at the UNSC session took note of these silences, reiterating the disproportionate impact of HIV on sub-Saharan Africa, the need for improved treatment access, and the larger context of underdevelopment in which the sub-Saharan pandemic is situated.[1] However, as in 2000, this HIV securitization produced no specific directives to address the regions and people most acutely impacted by HIV.

Expanded temporal scope

If Africa received less explicit attention, other aspects of the HIV-security nexus were considerably amplified in Resolution 1983. These amplifications include an expanded temporal focus to include post-conflict periods, and extensive discussion of gender and sexual violence. In both cases, the functional consequence is an expansion of UN authority, and authorization of deeper international incursions into states and bodies.

The ASCI report found little evidence to support the claim that HIV risk was most acute during conflict. Rather than prompting the authors to question the linkage between HIV and security, this instead produced the reformulated position "that HIV risks may be exacerbated during the transition from crisis or conflict to post-conflict situations" (de Waal et al., 2010, p. 65). While statements to this effect are repeated throughout the report, there is little supporting evidence provided. The position instead seems mainly rooted in the recognition that sexual violence continues to affect women in peacetime, and a resulting assumption that where rates of sexual violence are high, so too is the risk that this may be a vector for HIV transmission. (This point is discussed in the following section – Gender and sexual violence.)

The assertion that post-conflict peacebuilding should include HIV programming is reasonable. However, positioning this as something that should fall within the remit of HIV and security programming (as opposed to longer-term development or social justice work to address gender inequities and sexual violence) has the effect of expanding the scope of HIV and security as a policy and programming area, and consequently, expanding the authority of HIV and security practitioners into peacebuilding and transition periods where peacekeepers may no longer be present.

As a further example of this shifting locus of authority, Resolution 1308 positioned testing, counselling, and treatment as member state responsibilities. In contrast, Resolution 1983 positions this work within the UN's scope of authority, rather than devolving responsibility entirely to member states. Again, not only is programming expanded, but UN rather than state actors are directed to take on a larger role in that programming. By expanding UN authority in this way, greater IO reach into state practices is authorized, and matters previously considered domestic responsibilities are at least partially shifted to international actors.

By expanding the scope of HIV and security work to include DDR and SSR activities, the latter of which can extend for many years after the cessation of armed conflict, the authority of global HIV and security actors is extended over a longer period of time and expanded to encompass populations beyond uniformed services. The end result is deeper international reach into domestic matters, and into civilian populations. HIV and security programming has now expanded temporally into post-conflict (DDR) periods, expanded in population reach to include irregular armed forces (ex-combatants and militia) and civilian women, and expanded in programming scope to encompasses peer education training, behaviour interventions, improving access to services and assisting ex-combatants in transitions to civilian life (Cindy, 2010).

Gender and sexual violence

While Resolution 1308 made no explicit mention of gender, Resolution 1983 makes several references to gender (albeit understood as "women and girls", with seemingly no understanding that work with peacekeepers – assumed to be male – was also gendered work aimed at influencing presumed norms of masculine behaviour). Resolution 1983 is especially concerned with sexual violence as a manifestation of gender inequity that contributes to HIV transmission. Consequently, the initially narrow mandate of HIV prevention for peacekeepers is now linked to more expansive mandates to incorporate gender equity and sexual violence prevention into peacebuilding. While this is a high-level directive for coordination between UN staff working on gender and sexual violence and those working on HIV and security, it also constitutes an expansion of HIV and security actors' mandate. Furthermore, by expanding the populations meant to be targeted by HIV and security programming from peacekeepers to civilian women and girls in conflict and post-conflict situations, HIV and security actors are given authority to work with a much larger population than they were originally authorized to work with in Resolution 1308.

Even as there was amplified attention to sexual violence as a contributing factor to the spread of HIV, by 2011 peacekeepers were no longer considered to be perpetuators of this sexual violence. The UNSC sessions in 2000 largely characterized peacekeepers as dangerous vectors for HIV transmission. Resolution 1983, closely tracking ASCI report framings, instead positions peacekeepers as educators. UNSC session participants in 2011 spoke of the positive contribution peacekeepers could make to HIV prevention and education programming, rather than the threat they posed due to undisciplined sexual behaviours. Secretary-General Ban Ki-moon, for example, observed that

> before Resolution 1308 (2000) was adopted, uniformed personnel were viewed in terms of the [HIV] risk they might pose to civilians. Now we understand that United Nations troops and police are part of prevention, treatment and care. For example ... the United Nations Operation in Côte d'Ivoire and United Nations cosponsors are training troops and police on

HIV, human rights and gender equality. They are also providing technical support on HIV in disarmament, demobilization and reintegration (DDR) programmes.

(United Nations Security Council, 2011, p. 4)

The Executive Director of UNAIDS, Michel Sidibé, concurred, saying:

[W]e have come to understand that peacekeepers and the millions of people in uniform can play a leading role in HIV issues, as they secure peace around the world. Their extensive contacts with populations in conflict, post-conflict and other settings position them as agents of positive change, particularly with respect to preventing violence against women and girls in conflict.

(United Nations Security Council, 2011, p. 6)

In repositioning peacekeepers as educators, the boundaries demarcating who is threatened and who is threatening are shifted. Peacekeepers are brought into the realm of that which must be secured and protected (and can in turn secure and protect others), while perpetrators of sexual violence become the new threats, doubly dangerous to civilian women as they pose the threat of both sexual violence and HIV. What is left unexamined in these statements, and in Resolution 1983 itself, is who exactly *are* the perpetrators of sexual violence; there is no acknowledgement that some UN peacekeepers have themselves been the perpetrators of sexual violence, exploitation and abuse (Coomaraswamy, 2015, pp. 146–150). Neither is it clear exactly how peacekeepers will now prevent violence against women and girls, or, for that matter, how they will prevent HIV transmission in their role as educators.[2]

This re-imagined role of peacekeepers is perhaps the starkest example of the inversion of an argument used to securitize HIV in 2000. Peacekeepers, here, are discursively reconstructed from threats to educators, with a different set of shared characteristics and normative ascriptions. Functionally and normatively, peacekeepers in Resolution 1308 and Resolution 1983 are conceived of in entirely different and incompatible terms. Consequently, the content and meaning of 'HIV is a security threat' is transformed: HIV is no longer a threat located within the bodies and behaviour of peacekeepers, but is now (rather amorphously) a threat in post-conflict environments. The referent object is also transformed. In 2000, HIV was positioned as a threat to the stability of high prevalence states, to the combat-readiness of troops, and therefore to the effectiveness of UN peacekeeping operations. Resolution 1983 still acknowledges that HIV may threaten peacekeeping operations, but the putative threat to state stability is not the focus of this resolution. Instead, most of the resolution focuses on the threat that HIV poses to women and girls, especially via sexual violence.

Changing the referent object from states and peacekeeping operations to women and girls may seem a progressive move towards a human security framework. However, the source of the threat has also subtly shifted: it is now sexual violence and not HIV itself that is understood as the ultimate source of HIV threat. It is first of all not clear from the text of Resolution 1983 who the perpetrators of sexual violence are, nor how HIV education (or peacekeepers) will prevent sexual violence. More important, though, is the implicit message that if sexual violence were to be prevented, so too would HIV transmission. While preventing sexual violence would obviously improve the lives of women, girls and communities, by reducing the complex HIV vulnerabilities of women and girls to a problem of sexual violence, the security response to HIV remains truncated, in spite of the shift in referent object. It ignores, first, that in both conflict and peacetime, women additionally contract HIV through consensual relationships, albeit relationships embedded in structures that produce gendered, racialized, and socioeconomic disparities. When sexual violence becomes the focal point for interventions to prevent HIV, the myriad consensual routes of HIV transmission recede into the background, as do the gendered structural arrangements producing uneven power dynamics in these sexual relations. In short, preventing sexual violence is necessary, but not sufficient, to address complex gendered vulnerabilities to HIV (Seckinelgin, 2012). Furthermore, a focus on preventing HIV by preventing sexual violence continues to place the treatment and other needs of women already living with HIV largely outside the security response to HIV. And finally, positioning sexual violence as especially endemic to conflict and immediate post-conflict periods downplays the extent to which women and girls routinely experience violence in peacetime, in stable, well-functioning states – that is, it reduces women and girls' vulnerabilities to sexual and other forms of patriarchal violence to a problem driven by features of conflict and post-conflict environments.[3]

Expansion of programming

Resolution 1983 and the ASCI report endorsed significant expansion of HIV-related programming. The most divisive aspects of this expanded programming continue to be HIV testing and treatment, which remain contentious and unresolved.

Although the locus of perceived HIV threat has shifted away from peacekeepers' bodies, greater incursions into their bodies are now recommended (by the ASCI report) and authorized (by Resolution 1983). The ASCI report argues that HIV prevention in armed forces should be

> a departure from the individual-centred approach that has long been the norm for civilian HIV and AIDS policies and programs.... [U]tilizing the army's own established mechanisms for controlling the behaviour of individual soldiers has yielded greater results than individually oriented HIV prevention efforts by medical staff.... The core principle of the command-centred approach – that the primary responsibility for the health of military units lies with the military command, not the individual soldier or the military medical service – is compatible with either mandatory or voluntary testing for HIV.
>
> (de Waal et al., 2010, pp. 37–39)

The report concedes that the ethical and human rights implications of mandatory testing should be considered, particularly where treatment access is limited (de Waal et al., 2010, p. 39). But the command-centred approach it endorses, by making military command rather than individual soldiers responsible for the care and discipline of soldiers' bodies, effectively privileges the exigencies of military structures before and above the rights of individuals in those structures.

In the report's endorsement of a command-centred approach that could equally include mandatory or voluntary testing, debate is largely circumvented, and the potentially severe repercussions individuals might face as a result of testing HIV-positive are downplayed. The deferral of debate, and acceptance that the rights of some populations must be curtailed in order to protect the security of others, are both a hallmark of securitization. What is especially striking is that endorsement of a command-centred approach to HIV prevention and testing, which increases power over uniformed services members' bodies, has occurred even as those bodies are no longer understood as threats – that is, at a moment when the putative threat posed by peacekeepers has become less acute, and when an urgent, intrusive response should no longer, according to securitization theory, be warranted.

Although reach into bodies and territories to *test* for HIV is intensified through the endorsement of a command-centred approach, *treatment* reach in the security response to HIV has not undergone similar intensification, even though Resolution 1983 does include treatment in the list of services that can be incorporated "as appropriate" into in-mission HIV programming. Furthermore, although the referent object of the HIV security threat is now women and girls, and sexual violence prevention is meant to protect women and girls, this has the effect of making prevention of sexual violation, rather than provision of HIV treatment, central to threat response.

Everyday exceptionalism: securitized response through desecuritized structures

The robust promotion of prevention and testing has entrenched exceptionally deep bureaucratic reach into peacekeepers' bodies, even though those bodies are no longer understood as the source of HIV threat. The extent, nature and duration of IO reach into other populations has likewise expanded. At the same time, the bodies and lives of HIV-affected populations outside of peacekeeping missions remain largely free from securitized interventions – particularly from treatment access and other life-saving bodily incursions, which remain largely outside of the security response to HIV.

This expansion of HIV and security programming has become a form of everyday exceptionalism wherein a securitized response, characterized by exceptionally but selectively intrusive reach of international actors into territories and bodies, is now delivered in and through the desecuritized bureaucratic apparatus of UN implementing agencies. These include agencies whose primary mandate is not the maintenance of international security; they are also agencies whose work takes place largely outside of the public eye. These bureaucratic structures, part of the ostensibly rule-governed realm of normal politics, have actually become structures through which the rule-breaking action that characterizes securitization becomes both less visible and more expansive. Initially exceptional programming practices authorized by securitization become normalized over time as they are gradually enfolded into everyday bureaucratic practices. This programming also deepens and expands, abetted by the expansionist tendencies of bureaucracies as well as the good intentions of their staff.

The observations that HIV and security actors' authority has incrementally expanded, and that HIV and security has emerged as a discrete area of policy and programming expertise within bureaucratic structures, are not theoretically novel. Barnett and Finnemore (2004) have documented the tendency of IO authority to expand over time, while the CS concurs that securitization can become institutionalized over time (Buzan, Wæver, & de Wilde, 1998, p. 27) and its interlocutors have well established that securitization is enacted through everyday bureaucratic practices through which security actors affirm and expand their authority (Aradau, 2006; Bigo, 2000; McDonald, 2008; Neal, 2006; Salter & Piché, 2011; Williams, 2011).

The importance of everyday exceptionalism is mainly empirical: it helps us to trace the longer-term *consequences* of the bureaucratization of securitization, especially that the logic of securitization continues to shape the security response to HIV even as it increasingly settles into desecuritized bureaucratic structures and modes of programme delivery, and even as the meaning of 'HIV is a security threat' has evolved and inverted over time. That is, certain exceptional features of securitization are evident *even within* what at first glance may seem a desecuritized response: first, exceptional incursions into bodies and territories have continued; and second, work remains temporally, geographically and substantively bounded in ways that exclude many of the highest-prevalence southern African states that are neither hosts of nor major troop contributors to UN peace operations. The inside/outside and threatened/threatening boundaries constructed through securitization are maintained, and these divisions shape resulting programming. The exclusionary logic of securitization thus structures programming long after the initial moment of securitization has passed, and deeply institutionalizes rule-breaking and norm-violating work in bureaucratic structures.

Learning in securitization theory and security practice

We can now turn to the question of how the bureaucratic realm of policy and programming expertise occupied by HIV and security experts emerged, how and why these experts transformed the meaning of 'HIV is a security threat' from 2000 to 2011, and what this suggests about the role of actor learning in securitization processes. 'HIV and security' emerged as an area of academic, policy and programme expertise precisely through and as a result of securitization efforts. HIV securitization processes, that is, constructed the academic and the UN experts who now claim authority over the HIV-security nexus. These experts, in turn, reconstructed and redefined the meaning of 'HIV is a security threat' as they learned from each other and from their own experiences implementing HIV and security programming.

May's (1992) typology of policy learning can usefully guide this analysis. He distinguishes between political learning, which entails learning about advocacy strategies, political feasibility and how to better advance policy objectives in a particular political environment (339–340); and policy learning, which he further divides into instrumental policy learning and social policy learning. The former involves learning about the effectiveness of policy instruments (336), while the latter "entails a new or reaffirmed social construction of a policy ... it involves a rethinking ... about fundamental aspects of a policy....The prima facie evidence for social learning consists of changes in fundamental aspects of a policy, including redefined objectives ... [and] changes in target groups" (337–338). All three of these forms of learning are evident in actors' explanations of how and why they sought to change HIV and security policy and programming.

Actor learning and the changing meaning of 'HIV is a security threat'

In tracing the evolution of securitizing actors' thinking about HIV and security, two themes emerge: a continued belief in the power of security, coupled with acute awareness of the problematic aspects of the strategic invocation of security. Attempting to balance the potential benefits of invoking security with managing its sometimes undesirable consequences has been an ongoing and agonistic process for HIV and security actors. This continuous balancing act has contributed to the shifting meaning of 'HIV is a security threat', as actors have sought on the one hand to draw attention to HIV, but on the other, to downplay the sometimes damaging effects of presenting HIV as a uniquely threatening problem. This tension was neatly encapsulated by Peter Piot, who reflected on the power and danger of securitization strategies by observing

> it has pros and cons, afterwards I thought a lot about it. For example, it's [the UNSC] also the least democratic of all bodies in the UN. On the one hand that makes it a little more effective, or efficient.... So you exclude lots of countries that have something at stake, so that makes it the least democratic of all bodies. But it's a powerful body.... The lesson I think for other health issues is really that if you want to put something on the agenda you need a strategy, and you need to play where the big issues are.
>
> (Piot, 2009)

Interviewees' insistence on the special power of security, and their recommendation that advocates for other social issues should likewise strategically invoke security to attract attention and resources, is a form of learning based on the perception (albeit, as discussed in Chapter 5, a perception that may confuse correlation with causation) that the UNSC sessions effectively drew attention and resources to HIV. This is a classic example of political learning (May, 1992) about the organizational location of power in the UN system: it resides in the UNSC, and can be accessed by speaking security. This can partly explain actors' continued desire to position HIV as a security problem, and therefore a legitimate matter for UNSC and especially P5 intervention. (It also has the effect of perpetuating the structural power of traditional security actors, since it reaffirms the power of security rather than seeking to reorder political priorities such that HIV or other health issues, *rather than* security, are seen as having greater claim on resources. This is discussed in Chapter 7).

HIV securitization initially entailed a formally narrow scope. This narrow focus was recognized by UNAIDS actors, from the outset, as a problematic feature of the emerging security response to HIV, and UNAIDS and other HIV and security practitioners in the UN have since been working to rectify this narrowness by promoting broader intersectoral work. A UNAIDS staff member, for example, spoke of the need to reposition the security response "just where things come together, you know, drug control, crime, violence against women, et cetera – so instead of addressing those things as silos ... we've been constantly recognizing this, and constantly trying to break down those barriers, but they constantly get re-erected" (Keith, 2009).

As discussed in Chapter 5, breaking down programme 'silos' is made difficult as a result of organizational division of labour in the UN system. Additionally, though, the logic of securitization has its own imperatives; even as actors see the need to pursue a broader, integrated approach to HIV prevention, certain restrictions of this logic are still evident. Specifically, Resolution 1983 connects HIV to other threat discourses, especially those of sexual violence. Sexual violence narratives fit neatly into the logic of securitization: here too there are clear binaries of threatened and threatening, victims ("women and girls") and perpetrators, good and bad, inside and outside. The complexities of treatment access, structural reform, and redistributive projects remain outside of this simple binary logic and are not easily integrated into threat discourses. While securitizing agents learned that HIV prevention requires strategic integration and alignment with other issues, the possibilities for integration remain inherently limited by virtue of the binary nature of securitization logic and its reliance on discourses in which threat plays a central role.

Efforts to connect HIV to broader issues of gender and sexual violence in conflict have likewise, to some observers, had limited effect:

> Gender issues are still very much neglected or ignored.... Look at who's getting this, who's dying, who's doing the care for others, all of that, it's a tremendous burden on women and girls.... We all thought we were being very clever to bring this into the security world and get more attention, but still, *still* there's not a serious attempt to look at some of that. Even on [Resolution] 1325, OK, there's a whole heck of a lot going on in terms of reporting ... but you know, in the latest peace talks in, wherever, you name it, did you see any women's groups involved? No.
>
> (June, 2010)

The Security Council has not followed up, it's not as though they have cared, it's like [Resolution] 1325, you pass a resolution in 2000 and then ten years later you come back to look at it and you realize that women have not been involved in peacemaking or peacekeeping at all. If you use the UNIFEM figures ... of all peacekeeping negotiations from 2000 to 2010, women have constituted 1.6% of the participants. So [Resolution] 1325 is virtually a dead letter ... [and] the UN has been an abysmal failure in the Congo ... *nothing's* worked around sexual violence and transmission of the virus... the UN simply did nothing about, or nothing that was discernible about protecting women from violence in a serious way.

(Lewis, 2011)

These interviewees have learned that the security field, in addition to having its own logic, is also deeply gendered: there are persistent ideas about which post-conflict participants 'count' as security actors, who can speak with authority about issues related to state-building and security, and who should participate in peacebuilding processes (Coomaraswamy, 2015). HIV and security has remained a highly masculinized sphere in spite of efforts to incorporate strategies to address women's vulnerabilities to sexual violence in conflict.

Interviewees' reflections on the current state of HIV and security programming also suggest learning about the contingent, short-term nature of securitization, which sits in tension with the longer time horizons and systems-level interventions needed to address a slow-moving disease with a complex social etiology. One interviewee, for instance, expressed concern that

there's a kind of unfortunate complacency right now.... There were a lot of kind of doomsday people, talking about how terrible things were going to be in India, and China, and Russia, and so then when it didn't turn out quite as bad as expected, people are saying, oh, well, OK, now there's care and treatment ... I think, unfortunately, a lot of donors are thinking, "Oh, well, the big emergency is over."

(June, 2010)[4]

In response to what actors learned about the inherently time-limited and 'siloed' scope of initial HIV and security responses, and the limited ability of these responses to address gendered vulnerability, we see in the ASCI report and Resolution 1983 an effort to tie the initially narrow security response to HIV to longer-term post-conflict peacebuilding and ongoing efforts to address gender and sexual violence. This is a form of social policy learning: it has influenced HIV and security actors to expand the temporal and geographic scope of HIV and security programming, to extend it more deeply into the bodies of peace-keepers, and to expand the range of target populations to include a much wider range of uniformed and civilian populations, with particular attention to women.

Learning pathways: tracing the production of security knowledge

In tracing *how* these actors learned, and especially *who* they learned from, three main learning pathways were evident. First was practitioners' experiential learning, often through their work in peacekeeping missions and humanitarian emergency response. A second learning pathway entailed bureaucratic actors learning from each other; in particular, Resolution 1325, an expansive resolution dealing with gender and peacebuilding that was passed several months after Resolution 1308, and subsequent advocacy relating to addressing gender and sexual violence in conflict, became a model for later efforts on the part of UN staff to broaden and deepen the scope of Resolution 1308 and HIV and security work. Finally, practitioners learned from academics, and vice versa, with each group citing the writing and practices of the other as evidence that HIV was a security threat.

Chapter 4 demonstrated that experiential learning powerfully shaped Holbrooke's and Piot's perception of HIV and the ways in which it might constitute a security threat. Actors involved in HIV and security programming continued to learn from similar first-hand experience. In particular, the concerted effort to reposition peacekeepers as educators resulted in part from actor learning about a problematic aspect of securitization in general – the tendency towards us/Other binaries, and the construction of threatening Others – and the specific manifestation of this tendency in HIV securitization, namely the construction of peacekeepers as threats. As one interviewee observed, "the danger was that the way it was written, even in 1308 ... it was kind of looking at militaries as a threat ... militaries and at peacekeepers as vectors, not as particular at-risk populations" (June, 2010).

For those with whom I spoke, the impetus for challenging and revising this construction of peacekeepers was rooted largely in first-hand experience and experiential learning. Several interviewees spoke about working closely with peacekeepers and uniformed services, and witnessing them doing good work in difficult circumstances:

> I really love working with uniformed services.... There are some pretty progressive and forward-looking military leaders around the world.
>
> (June, 2010)

> You know, it's one thing about giving peacekeepers a bad name, "they're all perpetrators [of sexual abuse and exploitation], they're all bad" et cetera, but when I was there in [west Africa], I saw the same peacekeeping contingents dig out roads, get out WFP [World Food Programme] trucks from the mud, transport pregnant women to hospitals. [Military] doctors who had brought medicines for their own contingents were giving medicine to host communities ... and pregnant women were coming for assistance, and for regular check-ups.
>
> [*Later in the same interview*:] Uniformed services, it's important to show their different roles. Yes, they can be perpetrators, but they are protectors,

also. And they are family members, they are peer educators, or peers, you know?

(Cindy, 2010)

A lot of these [peacekeepers] have worked very hard [in] very harsh, very difficult conditions, they are facing huge challenges, and I think that work needs to be given its due.

(Alex, 2010)

HIV and security practitioners' experiences interacting directly with peacekeepers did not align with the positioning of peacekeepers in Resolution 1308, and the resulting dissonance between rhetoric and experience drove their efforts to revise the policy positioning of peacekeepers.

Experiential learning became a means of connecting the multiple levels at which securitization is articulated and practiced, and at which learning about securitization takes place. Actors working in the service of states, the UN and the international community were prompted to reformulate the meaning of 'HIV is a security threat' at the level of the international partly as a result of experiences at the 'local' level of UN peacekeeping missions. This form of experiential learning draws attention to the role of first-hand experience in connecting securitizing speech and security practices, and its power to reshape both. The contrast between Holbrooke's encounters with peacekeepers, and the experiences of these practitioners, also draws attention to how differently first-hand experiences can be interpreted – and the significant consequences that different interpretations can have on how security threats are articulated. This form of learning is highly contingent on individual subjectivity, the elevation of personal experience to the level of evidence, and the reformulation of policy positions based on that evidence. It suggests the extent to which public policy can be shaped by personal experience, which needs to be considered as an evidence source when analysing the origins and evolution of policy problematiques.

Bureaucratic actors also learned from each other. Several interviewees contrasted programming mandated by Resolution 1308 with work mandated by Resolution 1325 and other strategies to address gender and sexual violence in conflict. While frustrated at the lack of progress in implementing gender and sexual violence-related resolutions, interviewees spoke approvingly of the attention that gender and sexual violence had received at the UNSC, especially relative to HIV. They noted the relatively large number of resolutions addressing gender and/in conflict, and stressed that Resolution 1325 had catalysed a greater range of programming than had 1308 (June, 2010; Keith, 2009; Lewis, 2011). Explicitly connecting the 'narrow' mandate of Resolution 1308 to the broader mandate of 1325 and other gender and conflict resolutions therefore struck some UN staff as an advantageous strategy to secure greater attention to HIV, and to do so in a manner that connected HIV and security to other issues and programming activities.

In Resolution 1983's efforts to tie HIV and security to broader mandates, we see evidence of securitizing actors' learning from the securitizing moves of others. That is, Resolution 1983's linkage of HIV and security to gender and sexual violence – issues perceived as now having greater traction than the spectre of dangerous peacekeepers spreading HIV – was prompted at least in part by bureaucratic actors who observed and learned from their colleagues' efforts to securitize gender and sexual violence. This affirms the importance of bureaucratic context in shaping securitizing moves: changes in the bureaucratic policy environment can prompt securitizing actors to employ new tactics, including grafting their issue onto other agendas that seem to be ascending in political importance.

Finally, practitioners and security theorists also learned from each other. Through this learning, and especially by invoking each other as experts, each group established their areas of expertise over time. This practice of mutual, reciprocal citations advanced practitioners' and analysts' authority (by suggesting that they had academic evidence and external validation to back up their position that HIV was a security threat) and the authority of the person or entity being cited (because the citation could in turn be used as evidence that the person or entity in question was recognized as an expert in their field, by other experts). It is largely through this process that HIV and security knowledge has been produced, and the field of HIV and security established as a unique field of expertise.

Barnett and Prins have traced the repeated citation of "factoids": "soft opinions that have hardened into fact" (Barnett & Prins, 2006, p. 363), including that rates of STIs are higher among military than civilian populations, that have been used to advance the idea that HIV might impinge on military effectiveness. In addition to the repetition of those tenuous epidemiological claims, the larger idea that HIV is a security threat has similarly been repeated and a supporting evidence base built up through citational practices wherein the statement 'HIV is a security threat' is asserted in one document, which itself is later cited as evidence of the threat posed by HIV although the *nature* of that threat has been constructed quite differently across documents.

First, Resolution 1308 itself was subsequently cited as evidence that HIV is a security threat. When asked what documents or evidence sources they used to persuade donors that HIV prevention work in uniformed services was necessary, one interviewee responded that "of course we used the resolution [1308] itself" (June, 2010). Similarly, Resolution 1308 has been widely cited in academic work as empirical evidence that HIV is a security threat.

More broadly, the securitizing moves of practitioners at one point in time have later been cited by academics as evidence of HIV's status as a security threat. This evidence has in turn been used by practitioners to justify HIV and security work. For example, one of the earliest academic works on HIV and security, written by Stefan Elbe, cautiously accepted initial claims about high HIV prevalence rates in national militaries, suggesting that HIV would likely impact the effectiveness of armed forces and might have strategic implications; it also provisionally accepted that peacekeepers were vectors for HIV transmission, and suggested that HIV could potentially contribute to state collapse if measures were not taken to stop its spread (Elbe, 2003). Elbe was careful to position this analysis as "an initial, exploratory 'think piece'" based on limited evidence (Elbe, 2003, p. 10), and the monograph concludes by warning that framing HIV as a security threat might contribute to increased stigma and discrimination (Elbe, 2003, p. 64). The monograph has since been referenced by HIV and security practitioners, including by ASCI report authors, in a manner that elides the nuance and complexity of Elbe's analysis: it is simply cited as evidence that HIV is a security threat, even though the *meaning* of 'HIV is a security threat' in the ASCI report, in Elbe's academic work, and its use in practice by HIV and security practitioners varies significantly.

The ASCI report makes selective use of Elbe's work, citing two of his early publications that tentatively accept the proposition that HIV is a security threat (Elbe, 2002, 2003), but not his later, more nuanced and critical work (see especially Elbe, 2006, 2008). Elbe's two early publications are cited in the ASCI report to support statements that soldiers may be more likely to have unprotected sex, and that rape in the context of genocidal violence in Rwanda contributed to high rates of HIV among rape survivors. Neither of these points are (a) central to Elbe's arguments in those publications, or (b) supported by Elbe's own primary research. Rather, they are claims he makes in passing, and supports with reference to an evidence base that Elbe himself cautioned was insufficient to support definitive claims about the security and strategic impact of HIV.

Furthermore, early work (including Elbe's) focused on national security aspects of HIV – that is, the threat HIV could pose to militaries and state stability in the context of conflict – but the ASCI report, which focuses primarily on HIV in the context of sexual violence and post-conflict transitions, still cites this early work as evidence that HIV is a security threat. The meaning of 'HIV is a security threat' has evolved over time, yet citational practices create the impression of consensus; older work is cited in support of the contemporary understanding of 'HIV is a security threat', though there is at best an imperfect alignment between the different meanings of the phrase across time and across documents. The result is a form of knowledge generation in which a reciprocal and iterative relationship between practitioners and academics, particularly evident in their citational practices, first produced and then maintained the field of HIV and security expert knowledge and authority.

Implications for actor learning in securitization theory

The analysis suggests a mutually constitutive relationship between theorists and practitioners, wherein together they produce social reality in the form of broadly agreed-upon understandings about security problems and solutions. This has implications for securitization theory. A foundational assumption of securitization theory is that security trumps all. The CS framework additionally asserts that "the security quality [of a given issue] is supplied by politics" (Buzan et al., 1998, p. 32) and "it is the [political] actor, not the analyst, who decides whether something is to be handled as an existential threat" (Buzan et al., 1998, p. 34).

That is, the CS asserts that, first, security analysts and securitizing actors are distinct categories of social actors, and second, that securitizing actors in international relations, not analysts in IR, determine when security problems are defined and accepted as such.

There are two difficulties with holding, in a single theory, the dual claims that security trumps all, and that actors but not analysts have a political role to play in determining what can and should be securitized. Both are illustrated by the empirical case of HIV securitization. The first problem relates to the social power of security. If the statement that security trumps all – an assertion repeated across several security theories and by almost all of my interviewees – is taken to be objectively true, then the CS can indeed be considered apolitical (though this objectivist stance would be at odds with the CS's constructivist ontology). But if the CS helps to construct social reality by asserting that security holds inherent power to trump all other issues, thereby suggesting to political and IO actors a blueprint for drawing increased attention to an issue, then securitization theory is inherently political. It cannot stand outside of politics and analyse securitization; its theorists are participants through their acceptance of the social power of security. In other words, the theory's acceptance that security trumps all naturalizes a social construction, presenting as fact something that (1) is actually an empirical proposition that may or may not hold true in all circumstances and (2) denies its own agentic power in constructing, not simply reflecting, social reality. The theory is inherently political because it makes a claim about the utility of a specific political strategy (securitization) to achieve exceptional ends. The CS presents a political judgement – a claim about the strategic efficacy of invoking security – as a merely descriptive statement.

A second and closely related problem is the contention that there is a meaningful distinction between security actors and security analysts, and between the construction of and analysis of security problems. Given the extent to which the populations of securitizing actors and securitizing analysts have overlapped in HIV and security analysis, the actor/analyst and practice/theory distinction does not hold in this case (nor, others have argued, can it hold more widely (Aradau, 2004; Biersteker, 2010)). The production of the ASCI report is precisely an instance wherein

> [t]he securitisation analyst in writing … about a particular social reality is in part responsible for the co-constitution of this very reality, as by means of her own text this reality is (re)produced…. In writing or speaking security, the securitisation analyst herself executes a speech act.
>
> (Floyd, 2010, p. 47)

Jennifer Klot and Alex de Waal, for example, were lead authors of the ASCI report, and are routinely consulted by HIV and security practitioners in and beyond the UN. de Waal additionally holds an academic post, and both he and Klot are part of a densely interconnected network of researchers and practitioners that spans universities, research institutes, governments and multilateral organizations, including the UN. When they affirm in the ASCI report that HIV is a security threat, and describe what sort of threat it is, they do not reflect an already-established political consensus; rather, they participate in a reflexive, iterative dialogue between academics, practitioners and policy makers in which all parties contest and debate the meaning and political significance of the idea 'HIV is a security threat'. They are both analysts and actors.

Similarly, when HIV and security practitioners read the ASCI report and other policy documents citing de Waal, Elbe and other academics, they become the audience for academic claims (often drawing on securitization theory) about how and if HIV is a security threat – and for particular interpretations of those claims, which may not always fully reflect the nuance and complexity of the original academic research. Practitioners then evaluate these claims and use them as the basis for further securitizing moves and practices. While academics and practitioners may have different social *locations* in universities and IO bureaucracies, they are performing, together, the same social *function* of knowledge generation and construction of HIV as a security threat. It might then be most accurate to conceptualize this as a single epistemic community of securitizing actors, with mutually supporting academic and programmatic branches.

Moreover, even in policy areas beyond HIV, where there may be less overlap between the actors who securitize and the analysts who study securitizations, in setting out the criteria by which a securitization is judged as successful or not, academics do more than observe social reality when they compare empirical events to theoretical frameworks. They also evaluate, and on the basis of their evaluation of a securitization's success or failure, rightness or wrongness, they lend the weight of expert authority to political deliberations. Their conclusions in turn hold the potential to influence further political deliberations, and to influence the decision of other political actors to accept or reject a given securitization. As Watson (2012, p. 295) has also argued, establishing the assessment criteria used to determine whether a securitization is successful or is merely a securitizing move is itself a value-laden and political process.

If securitization theory has influenced 'real-world' security practice, the reverse is also true: security practice in international relations has shaped security studies in IR. Perhaps the most telling example of this is the repetition of the claim 'HIV is a security threat' in academic work, a claim that only appeared after 2000 and was catalysed by Resolution 1308. As discussed earlier, the claim that HIV is a security threat was largely, if cautiously, accepted by the earliest IR theorists to engage with the HIV-security nexus, and only later did more critical perspectives emerge. In other words, practitioners' strategic positioning of HIV, and claims about causal relationships between HIV prevalence and insecurity, have significantly influenced academic understandings of the relationship between HIV and security, and the trajectory of academic research agendas in this area.

Because actors and analysts learn from each other, and reformulate securitizations based on what they have learned, the content and meaning of a given securitization is not fixed at the moment of a securitizing speech act or through repetition of security practices. Rather, meaning is dynamic and changes over time. Securitizations and the meaning of a given threat construction (in this case 'HIV is a security threat') are unstable, continuously contested and reformulated based on what actors have learned from each other and from their own experiences. This learning process, moreover, reflects not only what actors learn about the threat itself, but also what they learn about their own political and organizational environment and the strategic securitizing moves most likely to achieve results within that context. This reaffirms that securitization is best understood theoretically and studied empirically as a process of constructing social reality that unfolds over time, and in which the content and meaning of a given securitization is treated as dynamic and emergent, not fixed.

Conclusion

The idea 'HIV is a security threat' has passed through the looking glass to form a set of inverted arguments that in some cases contradict those initially used to securitize HIV, but are nevertheless used to justify continued treatment of HIV as a security threat. While HIV itself remains securitized – the security response to HIV continues to entail transgression of territorial and bodily boundaries, and this has expanded since the initial securitizing moment – the structures and mechanisms through which this response is being executed are now those of routine bureaucratic politics. This 'everyday exceptionalism', wherein a securitized response is delivered through desecuritized mechanisms and structures, is evidence of the extent to which securitization logic continues to shape HIV and security programming long after the initial securitized moment has passed, and of the ways in which securitization and desecuritization are relational processes, entangled together on a single Möbius strip.

Another entangled, relational process involves the dense interconnections between the securitizing actors, practitioners and academics who have, together, come to constitute an epistemic community of HIV and security experts. Examining how and from whom securitizing actors learned over time suggests at least three learning pathways through which security knowledge is continually produced: practitioners learn through first-hand experience; bureaucratic actors learn from each other; and international relations actors learn from IR academics. These learning pathways can help us trace both why and how the content or meaning of a securitization evolves over time. Particularly with respect to the latter form of learning, this additionally illustrates that securitization, and social reality in international politics more broadly, is co-constituted by academics and practitioners – and further, that academic/practitioner categories are not always distinct. In the case of HIV securitization, the dense web of reciprocal citations and interconnections between academics and practitioners has effectively produced a single epistemic community of securitizing actors in which IR analysis influences international relations practices, and vice versa. This illuminates a political tension in securitization theory: if we accept the constructivist ontological premises of the CS, then we must also recognize that securitization theorists are inevitably implicated in the production of social reality and (security) knowledge about that social reality. This raises a complex set of questions about the politics of and in securitization theory, which are taken up in the next chapter.

Notes

1 As in 2000, some African states participating in the debate (Nigeria and South Africa) chose to have political leaders, rather than ambassadors, address the UNSC. Whereas these states sent their health ministers in 2000, in 2011 they sent more senior officials (the president of Nigeria and deputy president of South Africa). No global North states sent political leaders to the debate in 2011.
2 The positioning of peacekeepers as HIV educators may also be a wildly optimistic overestimation of their capacities. A 2007 survey of peacekeepers deployed to Haiti found limited knowledge of HIV despite high levels of HIV training coverage (Loche & Gurung, 2007), raising questions about the extent to which even those who have received HIV education have the requisite knowledge and skills to serve as peer educators.
3 Additionally, "women and girls" continue to be understood as a population separate and distinct from peacekeepers, uniformed services and combatants, who are assumed to be male; women and girls are understood to be in need of protection from sexual violence, but not themselves the perpetrators of violence. MacKenzie (2010) argues that these gendered assumptions can result in approaches wherein, even when women are identified as a population of special concern, female combatants' needs may not be recognized or appropriately addressed. Kirby (2015) additionally observes that such framings overlook that men and boys can also be victims of sexual violence.
4 On the effect of 'end of emergency' perspectives, see also Ingram (2013).

References

Alex (2010, 12 April). (Personal interview with author).

Aradau, Claudia. (2004). Security and the democratic scene: desecuritization and emancipation. *Journal of International Relations and Development*, 7(4), 388–413.

Aradau, Claudia. (2006). Limits of security, limits of politics? A response. *Journal of International Relations and Development*, 9(1), 81–90.

Barnett, Michael & Finnemore, Martha. (2004). *Rules for the World: International Organizations in Global Politics*. Ithaca, NY: Cornell University Press.

Barnett, Tony & Prins, Gwyn. (2006). HIV/AIDS and security: fact, fiction and evidence – a report to UNAIDS. *International Affairs*, 82(2), 359–368.

Biersteker, Thomas J. (2010). Interrelationships between theory and practice in International Security Studies. *Security Dialogue*, 41(6), 599–606.

Bigo, Didier. (2000). When two become one: internal and external securitisations in Europe. In Morten Kelstrup & Michael C. Williams (Eds.), *International Relations Theory and the Politics of European Integration: Power, security and community* (pp. 171–204). New York: Routledge.

Buzan, Barry, Wæver, Ole, & de Wilde, Jaap. (1998). *Security: A New Framework for Analysis*. Boulder, CO: Lynne Rienner.

Cindy (2010, 31 March). (Personal interview with author).

Coomaraswamy, Radhika, et al. (2015). *Preventing Conflict, Transforming Justice, Securing the Peace: A Global Study on the Implementation of United Nations Security Council Resolution 1325*. New York: UN Women.

de Waal, Alexander. (2003). How will HIV/AIDS transform African governance? *African Affairs*, *102*(406), 1–23.

de Waal, Alexander. (2006). *AIDS and Power: Why There Is No Political Crisis – Yet.* New York: Zed Books.

de Waal, Alexander, Klot, Jennifer E., Mahajan, Manjari, Huber, Dana, Frerks, Georg, & M'Boup, Souleymane. (2010). *HIV/AIDS, Security and Conflict: New Realities, New Responses.* New York: AIDS, Security and Conflict Initiative (Social Science Research Council & Netherlands Institute of International Relations Clingendael).

Elbe, Stefan. (2002). HIV/AIDS and the changing landscape of war in Africa. *International Security*, *27*(2), 159–177.

Elbe, Stefan. (2003). *Strategic Implications of AIDS* (Vol. Adelphi Paper 357). Oxford: Oxford University Press.

Elbe, Stefan. (2006). Should HIV/AIDS be securitized? The ethical dilemma of linking HIV/AIDS and security. *International Studies Quarterly*, *50*(1), 199–144.

Elbe, Stefan. (2008). Risking lives: AIDS, security and three concepts of risk. *Security Dialogue*, *39*(2–3), 177–198.

Floyd, Rita. (2010). *Security and Environment: Securitisation Theory and US Environmental Security Policy.* New York: Cambridge University Press.

Garrett, Laurie. (2005). *HIV and National Security: Where Are the Links?* New York: Council on Foreign Relations.

Ingram, Alan. (2013). After the exception: HIV/AIDS beyond salvation and scarcity. *Antipode*, *45*(2), 436–454.

June (2010, 23 April). (Personal interview with author).

Keith (2009, 27 October; 18 November). (Personal interview with author).

Kirby, Paul. (2015). Ending sexual violence in conflict: the Preventing Sexual Violence Initiative and its critics. *International Affairs*, *91*(3), 457–472.

Lewis, Stephen (2011, 17 January). (Personal interview with author).

Loche, Elisabeth & Gurung, Dr. Megh. (2007). *HIV/AIDS Knowledge, Attitude and Practice Survey: UN Uniformed Peacekeepers in Haiti.* New York: United Nations Department of Peacekeeping Operations (DPKO) Peacekeeping Best Practices Section.

MacKenzie, Megan. (2010). Securitization and de-securitization: female soldiers and the reconstruction of women in post-conflict Sierra Leone. In Laura Sjoberg (Ed.), *Gender and International Security: Feminist Perspectives* (pp. 151–167). New York: Routledge.

May, Peter J. (1992). Policy learning and failure. *Journal of Public Policy*, *12*(4), 331–354.

McDonald, Matt. (2008). Securitization and the construction of security. *European Journal of International Relations*, *14*(4), 563–587.

McInnes, Colin. (2006). HIV/AIDS and security. *International Affairs*, *82*(2), 315–326.

McInnes, Colin & Rushton, Simon. (2013). HIV/AIDS and securitization theory. *European Journal of International Relations*, *19*(1), 115–138.

Neal, Andrew W. (2006). Foucault in Guantánamo: towards an archaeology of the exception. *Security Dialogue*, *37*(1), 31–46.

Piot, Peter (2009, 23 October). (Personal interview with author).

Rushton, Simon. (2010). AIDS and international security in the United Nations system. *Health Policy and Planning*, *25*, 495–504.

Salter, Mark B. & Piché, Geneviève. (2011). The securitization of the US–Canada border in American political discourse. *Canadian Journal of Political Science*, *44*(4), 929–951.

Seckinelgin, Hakan. (2012). *International Security, Conflict and Gender: "HIV/AIDS is Another War".* New York: Routledge.

United Nations Security Council. (7 June 2011). *Resolution 1983 (2011)*. (S/RES/1983 (2011) – adopted by the Security Council at its 6547th meeting, 7 June 2011).

United Nations Security Council. (2011). Transcript: Agenda: Maintenance of international peace and security: impact of HIV/AIDS epidemic on international peace and security (United Nations Security Council, 66th year, 6547 meeting, Tuesday 7 June 2011, S/PV.6547).

Watson, Scott D. (2012). "Framing" the Copenhagen School: integrating the literature on threat construction. *Millennium: Journal of International Studies, 40*(2), 279–301.

Whiteside, Alan, de Waal, Alexander, & Gebre-Tensae, Tsadkan. (2006). AIDS, security and the military: a sobering appraisal. *African Affairs, 105*(419), 201–218.

Williams, Michael C. (2011). The continuing evolution of securitization theory. In Thierry Balzacq (Ed.), *Securitization Theory: How Security Problems Emerge and Dissolve* (pp. 212–222). New York: Routledge.

7 The limits of 'securing' health through securitization

Careful empirical consideration of the UNSC's securitization of HIV from origins to outcomes suggests that it effected little change in the global response writ large; that Africa, the continent whose pandemic was the ostensible reason for this securitization, has been at once deeply implicated but largely invisible in the securitized response to HIV; that this response, even as it expanded, has not incorporated robust treatment access, or reached those most vulnerable to and at risk of HIV, especially civilian women in southern Africa; and that within this response, human rights have been displaced and deferred, especially with respect to testing and treatment for UN peace mission staff. Moreover, this has been the case in spite of the aims of (some of) the architects of HIV securitization to catalyse significant change in the global response, and concerted efforts on the part of securitizing actors to revise and reinterpret the meaning of 'HIV is a security threat' over time, in the enduring hope of effecting progressive change. This chapter therefore develops the normative critique towards which the previous chapters have been building: that securitization cannot 'secure' health, and is inherently limited as a transformative social justice strategy.

As well as the political implications of this analysis, it has theoretical and normative implications for theories of security, including securitization, that frequently *assume* security (1) trumps all and (2) draws attention and resources to an issue, when these are actually empirical propositions to be tested – and when, as I and others (Rushton, 2010) have argued, neither proposition held true in this case. There is also an implicit assumption in much securitization theory and international relations practice that securitization, with its power to catalyse rapid, decisive action, produces effective if illiberal outcomes. Yet HIV securitization in the UN system challenges this assumption, as it did not significantly improve treatment access or mitigate the African pandemic, both of which had been central aims of securitizing actors. More insidiously, these assumptions are all predicated on the acceptance that security is and should be the top political priority, rather than posing a deeper critique of the 'normal' political and social order that produces and supports this hierarchy of political priorities. This tacit acceptance of the special power of security is especially problematic if, as suggested in Chapter 6, analysts' production of security knowledge holds the potential to shape social reality. But neither the empirical limitations of securitization as a political strategy, nor the presence of some problematic theoretical assumptions about security, mean that securitization theory is inherently unable to support normative analysis or social justice praxis. On the contrary, securitization theory can and should be used to question and critique the foundational assumptions driving 'real world' securitizations, and to support normative and critical projects.

To develop this argument, the chapter begins by summarizing what the book's empirical analysis has suggested about how, and in what ways, securitization appears inherently limited as a transformative political strategy. It then considers what security-in-use – that is, how the word 'security' was actually used and understood by actors in this instance – might suggest about limits not only to securitization, but more generally to the invocation of security in social justice strategies. It does so on the basis that claims about what security can and cannot do or mean, in theory, must ultimately be assessed against empirical attempts to shift the meaning of security and to invoke it to achieve social justice goals. The chapter then asks, in light of these limitations, what strategies beyond securitization might exist, and especially, what potential might exist in desecuritization techniques in which normal politics itself becomes the site and object of emancipatory praxis. In particular, the chapter suggests that the securitization as policy process framework can usefully support precisely this type of critique.

The question of what might exist beyond securitization is especially important at a moment when HIV is increasingly regarded as a problem no longer justifying exceptional response and funding (Ingram, 2013), and when there are growing calls for HIV to be 'normalized' or 'integrated' into broader sexual and reproductive health programming and health systems strengthening efforts (Whiteside & Smith, 2009). We of course need to be cautious in stating that HIV is 'no longer exceptional': while maintaining high levels of HIV funding relative to funding for other health issues is increasingly challenging in a climate of austerity (Ingram, 2013), there are many aspects of the HIV response that continue to be characterized by exceptional *practices*. In addition to practices specifically associated with the UNSC's HIV securitization, which have been the focus of this book, other forms of exceptionalism include the criminalization of HIV transmission, which continues to result in the criminal prosecution and imprisonment of people living with HIV who have failed to disclose their sero-status to sexual partners (O'Byrne, Bryan, & Roy, 2013); travel restrictions barring entry of people living with HIV to some states; the continued exceptional stigma attached to HIV relative to other diseases; and emerging forms of surveillance and treatment adherence strategies.[1] Recalling the proposition that securitization and desecuritization can be understood as a Möbius strip in which one state bleeds into the other, these exceptional elements are another instance of the continuities that persist even into seemingly unexceptional or desecuritized politics. Nevertheless, to the extent that the global HIV response is in or approaching a period "after the exception" (Ingram, 2013), the political and analytical considerations, constraints and opportunities in this new landscape may be different than those evident when HIV was first securitized.

The limits of securitization

HIV securitization in the UN system entailed the establishment and maintenance of boundaries, both discursive (between threatened and threatening subjects), and organizational (for example, between humanitarian and security actors). These boundaries served to establish the limits of the security response to HIV, such that uniformed services and the security sector were folded into the response, but the people and states most affected by HIV were excluded. Within the security response, securitization catalysed rule-breaking, exceptionalism and transgression: the initial UNSC debates broke the rule that the UNSC's sole focus should be armed conflict, the resulting programming entailed exceptional reach into and influence over peacekeepers' bodily practices, and this reach gradually expanded to other populations and spaces, creating and normalizing what I have called 'everyday exceptionalism'. But the uniquely devastating impact of HIV in high-prevalence sub-Saharan African states, especially in southern Africa and especially among civilian women living in poverty, was gradually erased from this threat response, wherein security was conflated with and reduced to peacekeeping, and the policy response within the security field limited to testing and prevention strategies, not provision of ARVs or comprehensive care and support.

In sum, securitization has served to maintain boundaries and binaries which have in turn constrained the range of action possible within the security response to HIV. Four key limitations inherent in HIV securitization emerged through the book's empirical analysis: first, securitization did not and could not meaningfully address the structural drivers of HIV; second, its logic of threat construction and response relied on and perpetuated us/Other boundaries that preclude creation of inclusive political communities; third, it has been characterized by a fundamental instability; and fourth, in the context of the UN system, there were additionally enduring organizational constraints arising from entrenched definitions of security. Considering each of these in turn can illustrate how and why securitization was inevitably and inherently limited, from the outset, as a transformative strategy.

Securitization cannot address the structural drivers of HIV

Although treatment access was and remains a tremendous unmet need, and was explicitly raised as an urgent issue by participants in the 2000 UNSC sessions, HIV securitization in the UNSC had no direct effect on treatment access. I have already argued that this was a significant limitation of international HIV securitization. Yet even achieving universal treatment access, while it would be a tremendous accomplishment, would still not be sufficient by itself to halt or reverse the pandemic. As Barnett and Whiteside (2006, p. 369) argue, "ARTs, even at much lower prices, are not 'the answer'. They are part of an answer, which must include head-on confrontation with the conditions that contribute to the epidemic in the first place. Those conditions are poverty-related risk." Piot (2006, p. 529) similarly calls for tackling the structural drivers of this epidemic, especially sex inequality, stigma and discrimination around homosexuality and sexuality in general, and poverty and desperation in all their aspects. This challenge is perhaps the greatest of all those facing the AIDS response, given the pervasiveness of the barriers to life-protecting services to women, the socially marginalized, and the poor. No technological solution exists for overcoming them.

Addressing the structural drivers of HIV remains a political problem, not a technical one.

Of course this does not mean technological and medical solutions are unimportant; obviously advances in HIV treatment have had a tremendous positive impact. But treatment access remains uneven, with many people living with HIV, especially in sub-Saharan Africa, continuing to experience treatment access barriers: by the end of 2012, only 7.6 of 21.2 million eligible Africans were receiving ARV treatment (Joint United Nations Programme on HIV/AIDS (UNAIDS), 2013), and this had risen to only 10.6 million by the end of 2014 (Joint United Nations Programme on HIV/AIDS (UNAIDS), 2015).[2] Additionally, ARVs do not address the circumstances that make some populations especially vulnerable to HIV in the first place, and these circumstances are usually the same ones that make it especially difficult for those populations, if and when they contract HIV, to access treatment (Joint United Nations Programme on HIV/AIDS (UNAIDS), 2014).

Securitization did not and could not dislodge these structural drivers, precisely because its logic creates the imperative to protect one set of actors from another through defensive measures to contain or eradicate threat. As shown in Chapter 5, in the security response to HIV, the containment strategies of securitization have been devolved to the level of individual behaviour change interventions. Responsibility for policing and enforcing behaviour has partly shifted to military leadership through the endorsement of "command-centred" approaches, but prevention strategies remain targeted at the individual, not structural level. Securitization's threat response is rooted in the logic of containment, not structural change; it is inherently unequipped to address the structural drivers of HIV transmission.[3]

Securitization's logic is premised on exclusion

Securitization was additionally an inadequate means of transforming the global response or addressing structural drivers because its threat-based logic relies on us/Other binaries, which necessarily produce both difference and hierarchy. It is premised on exclusion: the protection of those inside relies on the exclusion and casting out of people and entities that, deemed to be threatening, are denied protection. I have argued in previous chapters that these boundaries, and the practices they authorize in the name of threat response, are constructed and maintained largely through ideas and discourse. Ideas about HIV are shaped by racialized, gendered discourses about threat, which then produce and institutionalize a threat response predicated on defense against the Other.

This logic becomes especially important when we consider the status of Africa in the UNSC sessions and resulting HIV and security programming intended to defend against the threat of HIV. We saw in Chapter 3 that the threat discourses enabling HIV securitization rested in large part on historically-produced, racialized and gendered discourses in which Africa and Africans were already produced as threatening Others. These threat discourses were evident in the speech acts that securitized HIV, particularly in the ambiguous status of Africa and Africans during the 2000 UNSC sessions, where the continent and its people were presented as both threatened and threatening. Ultimately, by the policy implementation stage there was an erasure of the continent as an explicit focus of programming interventions, and by 2011 Africa was not even mentioned in Resolution 1983. Yet despite the progressively decreasing visibility of Africa, programming in the UN's security response to HIV was predicated on, produced and preserved an African Other-ness. Predominantly African territories and bodies at once (1) became the targets of exceptional incursions through which rights were displaced and deferred, when they were 'inside' security by virtue of being implicated in peacekeeping; and (2) when they were 'outside' security by virtue of *not* being implicated in peacekeeping, became excluded from the security response, such that international HIV securitization excluded some of the most acutely affected populations and states.

The instability of securitization

The ambiguous status of Africa and its relation to HIV securitization points to a further limitation of securitization as a social justice strategy: it is characterized by a fundamental instability. The meaning of 'HIV is a security threat', and the question of how and to whom HIV is threatening have been a matter of vigorous debate. While Resolution 1308 attempted to fix a narrow interpretation of 'HIV is a security threat', identifying peacekeepers as threatening vectors of HIV transmission, and states and state stability as the referent object in need of protection, the idea continued to be contested and reinterpreted. By the time Resolution 1983 was passed, the referent object had shifted from states to women and girls, the source of the threat was identified as sexual violence and not peacekeepers, and peacekeepers themselves were now situated as educators.

Because securitization is an ongoing meaning-making process, the idea '[X] is a security threat' is never completely fixed, but is rather dynamic and evolves over time. Consequently, securitizations are inherently unstable, because a "logic of existential threat, survival and political realism can be indefinitely reversed to securitize other referent objects" (Aradau, 2004, p. 401). This instability could be regarded as a potential to be exploited: if an idea is open to reinterpretation, and referent objects can be changed, then could the meaning of 'HIV is a security threat' not be revised such that people living with HIV would become the population to be secured through provision of treatment and social supports?

Aside from the fact that this did not happen in the case of HIV securitization, in spite of the fact that Resolution 1983, the ASCI report and associated manoeuvring to redefine how and to whom HIV is threatening was undertaken with precisely this aim, the very instability that makes it possible to endlessly revise the meaning of '[X] is a security threat' also makes it unsuitable to achieve the enduring structural change that would be needed to address the structural drivers of HIV. Such change would require a degree of fixity and permanence in service delivery and redistributive mechanisms, which in turn implies relative stability in the underpinning ideas that define the populations for whom those services and mechanisms exist. Securitization, with its short time horizons, shifting meanings and capacity for infinite reversals, cannot create the stable ground upon which to accomplish this necessarily incremental, long-term change. Obviously, there is a point at which all ideas are inherently unstable. Ideas about who should benefit from redistributive strategies, and how, can and do evolve over time; this is not a limitation unique to securitization. However, in conjunction with its other limitations, the instability of securitization makes it especially problematic as a transformative strategy capable of producing enduring change.

Organizational constraints

Securitizing logic and policy directives were also interpreted through and reinforced by the specific organizational structures of the UN, in which security is already intersubjectively understood (and institutionalized) as national or human; in which security is equated with the security sector; and in which programming and jurisdictional authority are predicated on the distinction between security and humanitarian activities and actors. At the policy implementation stage, these organizational structures replicated, through bureaucratic practices and especially through boundary work, the logic of division, exclusion, exception and maintenance of us/them, inside/outside borders to define and delimit the security response to HIV. While this is less a limitation of securitization itself than of the organizational location of this specific securitization strategy, it nevertheless indicates another reason for caution in pursuing securitization as a means of transforming existing power relations and distribution of resources, especially at the international level. The UN is far from the only actor implicated in global health and global security, but it is nevertheless an important one; it would be difficult to imagine a global-level securitizing move in which no part of the UN system was implicated. Once brought into that system, anything labelled as 'security' will be subject to a similar process of boundary work to determine the appropriate location, lead agencies, and limits of a securitized response.

This too is not inevitable; it is in principle possible that the UN system could undergo structural change that might produce different institutional divisions of labour, a different delineation between security and other actors and organizational units, and therefore less conflation of security with the security sector, armed conflict and uniformed services. There is a point, however, at which path dependence makes this degree of organizational change unlikely. Certainly the number of failed attempts at UN reform (including UNSC reform that would dislodge the current P5 power structure and allocate greater authority to the global

South in matters having to do with international security) should temper any optimism that, in the short run, organizational structures and norms are likely to change to the extent that significantly new security definitions and practices could be institutionalized. Supporting this view, as discussed in Chapter 5, even the new UNAIDS unit created as a result of Resolution 1308 precisely to support integrated action on security and humanitarian responses to HIV, still maintained functional separation between security and humanitarian programming, and equated security with the security sector. This new unit accepted, rather than challenging, not just dominant organizational divisions of labour, but also an existing organizational logic of security and the structures through which this logic has been institutionalized.

Security-in-use and the practical limits of security

The organizational constraints of the UN system, particularly deeply institution-alized and widely accepted understandings of what security 'really' means, raise larger questions about whether, in addition to the limits of securitization, there might also be limits to invoking *security* as a social justice strategy.

This book has suggested that securitization is a dangerous strategy through which to 'secure' social change. Yet not all analysts would agree with this claim. Floyd (2007, 2011), for example, suggests that securitization can be just and eth-ically right, while Roe (2012) contends that securitization need not entail a 'neg-ative' logic. Beyond securitization theory, security-as-emancipation theorists (Basu, 2011; Booth, 1991, 2005; Nunes, 2012, 2014) would argue that a dif-ferent invocation of security could have produced quite different results, and that while *securitization* may be limited as a political strategy, this is not true of all invocations of security to achieve social change.[4] At the core of these distinct visions of what both securitization and security can and cannot do is a debate about whether or not security itself has a distinctive logic (see for example Balzacq, 2015).

These claims ultimately need to be adjudicated through contextualized empirical analysis (Browning & McDonald, 2011). Our theoretical claims about the logic of security, when used as the basis for assessing the utility of invoking security in social justice struggles, also need to confront actual instances when actors have explicitly invoked security and attempted to bend it to emancipatory ends. Analysis of security-in-use can tell us what 'security' as a word, concept and practice actually means to specific securitizing actors, and therefore what it can or cannot realistically be expected to achieve in a given context. If we follow the injunction of sociological variants of securiti-zation theory, which emphasize the importance of the specific, concrete polit-ical and organizational contexts within which securitizing moves occur (e.g. Balzacq, 2011; Bigo, 2005; Salter, 2008), we need to consider not only the logic of security, in the abstract, but also the empirics of security-in-use: beyond theoretical claims about what security might hypothetically be capable of doing, what did it *actually* do in this case?

I have argued that tracing security-in-use, that is, how 'security' was actually deployed and interpreted when HIV was securitized in the UN system, shows that efforts to place the bodily insecurity of people living with and vulnerable to HIV (especially Africans, and especially civilian women) at the centre of security discourse and practice, and efforts to link security to HIV treatment access, failed to dislodge deeply held organizational norms about what security 'really means'. Empirically, the word 'security', once invoked in the process of HIV securitization, immediately drew actors' attention to national security, the security sector and to peacekeeping, which then became the site for practices and programmes understood to comprise the defensive, containment-focused security response to HIV. I have further argued that the very discourses that made it pos-sible for HIV and Africa to be conjoined via securitizing speech themselves relied on historically-produced threat constructions in which HIV and Africa were always already placed in opposition to, not included within, the realm of that which needed to be secured. 'Speaking security' therefore moved HIV into the security sector and authorized exceptional interventions within that sector, but neither the security sector nor the global response writ large were trans-formed in ways that significantly benefited the majority of people living with or vulnerable to HIV.

This suggests that in practice, especially in the UN system, invoking security may risk ceding too much ground to those who have already claimed security and its associated structures for themselves, regardless of whether this invoca-tion is undertaken as a securitizing move or some other political strategy. The securitization of HIV represented a partial critique of extant political priorities, in that it recognized the perceived importance of security relative to other polit-ical concerns. But it entailed limited recognition of the extent to which the meaning and scope of 'security' programming, and actors with authority to address security concerns, had already been fixed in and through prior, very durable, organizational structures, practices and norms. Consequently, HIV secu-ritization ultimately reinforced what it began by critiquing: an existing set of political priorities in which security is (1) already, notwithstanding the presence of human security discourses, understood to refer mainly to national security and the security sector, and (2) considered more important than health.

Security-in-use, in this case, reveals the extent to which 'security', in the organizations and institutions of international politics, is deeply entwined with military, national security, and geopolitical concerns. This entanglement is evident at a deep, historically produced discursive level, and at the level of organizational, bureaucratic structures and practices. Both produce significant constraints to how security can be spoken, understood and enacted in policies and programmes. Of course, in principle, change is always possible; a socially constructed world can always be de- and re-constructed. But "the socially consti-tuted is often sedimented as structure and becomes ... relatively stable in prac-tice" (Buzan, Wæver, & de Wilde, 1998, p. 35). This was certainly evident in HIV securitization in the UN system, where actors tried unsuccessfully to achieve a social justice project – resource redistribution that would enable universal treatment access – in and through the discourses and structures of security. In this 'real world' scenario, the logic of security *was* the logic of securitization, and this logic failed to produce a transformed and transformative response to HIV.

Yet if HIV securitization in the UN system suggests the limits of securitization (and perhaps, any invocation of security) as a strategy to transform the global response, it equally suggests a tremendous failure on the part of normal politics and global public health actors both in and beyond the UN. Much of the initial impetus for HIV securitization arose from Piot's frustration with the obstructionism and infighting of UNAIDS' cosponsoring agencies, and with bureaucrats who placed the protection of their organizational turf over the welfare of the populations those organizations were created to serve. More broadly, it arose from the perception that global health actors and national ministries of health were collectively so ineffective and lacking political power that responsibility for addressing HIV needed to be taken away from health actors to produce an effective response. Actors' recourse to securitization strategies is also a strong critique of the health sector and of normal politics.

This presents a difficult question: if securitization did not catalyse the normative and political shift sought by Piot and others in the global response – and if, as I argue, it *cannot* produce such a shift – but the public health models of normal politics also fell far short of a transformative, socially just response, what other options might exist? One approach, espoused by security-as-emancipation theorists, is to transform the meaning of security itself. This approach, while situating emancipatory projects within security, does so from the premise that "the meaning of security is ultimately tied to the experience of being insecure" and, in somewhat circular logic, that "more security means the alleviation of the insecurities that are experienced by individuals and groups every day" (Nunes, 2014, p. 8). Other approaches suggest, in contrast, that emancipation or normative projects more generally are best sought through desecuritization strategies (Aradau, 2004; Hansen, 2012).

These do not of course exhaust the political options available to activists and practitioners, nor the theoretical approaches available to analysts. Outside of political science, the majority of HIV work (in both the academic and activist sense) has never situated itself in security politics or theory (Farmer, 2003; Fassin, 2007; Hunter, 2010; Mugyenyi, 2008; Nguyen, 2010; Patton, 1990). But my concern is specifically with the points at which HIV, security, and securitization strategies intersect, both in academic analysis and the political praxis of actors in the global response. HIV has, in the 'real world' of international politics, been securitized; the most sustained academic engagement with this securitization has been in and through various security theories; and as discussed elsewhere in this book, the dense interconnections between actors and analysts have created a situation in which both work together to produce knowledge about HIV and security which then shapes social reality. This knowledge production has had significant political consequences: the UNSC's return to HIV in 2011 was triggered by practitioners' efforts to promote continued securitization of HIV, which efforts they undertook in part because of (or, at a minimum, with the assistance of) academic analysis presented in the ASCI report recommending that HIV should continue to be treated as a security threat.

There is then theoretical and practical value in considering specifically how and in what ways the HIV-security nexus can be reimagined and remade, and especially how the logic and practice of securitization might be disrupted or undone. Therefore, with the proviso that this book has never intended to propose a definitive blueprint of how HIV (or security) politics ought to be conducted in the future, I turn now to the question of what, given the empirical limits of securitization as a transformative strategy, it might mean to pursue a desecuritization of HIV.

Desecuritization as transformation of normal politics

Recommending a turn to desecuritization may strike some readers as misguided: either because HIV continues to deserve an exceptional (Whiteside & Smith, 2009) and securitized (Elbe, 2009) response, or because desecuritization may still risk keeping us within the logic of security (Aradau, 2004), or because it risks silencing and overlooking the needs of desecuritized subjects (Hansen, 2012; MacKenzie, 2010) and perpetuating inequalities (Buzan et al., 1998, pp. 210–211), or because in theory security has no inherent logic and could potentially be made the basis for an emancipatory project in which health programming might become "a bridge for peace" (Nunes, 2014, p. 113). This section, then, begins by outlining why desecuritization is warranted (as well as considering the crucial question of what *type* of desecuritization is required in this case), before discussing how securitization theory, and the policy process model presented in this book, can support desecuritization efforts.

Why desecuritization

I have already suggested on empirical grounds (i.e. the ways in which security-in-use so readily directs actors back towards military and national security concerns and a focus on the security sector) that invoking security can be a dangerous strategy through which to achieve emancipatory ends. Situating emancipatory projects within security paradigms, regardless of how security is (re)defined in those paradigms, additionally makes these projects reliant on an objectivist assumption that security is inherently the highest of political goals. This tacit acceptance that security not only is but should be the most important of political priorities is troublingly deterministic insofar as it requires acceptance of this prioritization before any empirical political engagement. It is an oblique acceptance of a political order in which social justice objectives can only be achieved if recast as security problems. With the vast range of social and political expression available in the realm of normal politics, it is unclear to me why it should be preferable to pursue emancipation through redefinition of security, especially when this risks engaging structures and discourses that so easily conflate security with national security, militaries and the security sector. Equally, flattening the vast and varied terrain of human experience – and human suffering – by deeming it all and only a matter of insecurity seems to needlessly foreclose other forms of protest and resistance, truncating potential avenues of social and political change.

In the end, however, the suggestion that invoking security (whether in or beyond securitization strategies) seems to entail demonstrable dangers and limitations, and few certain benefits, is derived not from theoretical principles, but "reflexive and context-specific" (Browning & McDonald, 2011) empirical analysis. Thus, while realizing that security-as-emancipation theorists will disagree with these claims, I emphasize that the analysis is not intended to dispute their emancipatory political project, with which I am broadly aligned, nor to entirely dismiss their theoretical claims. I am merely observing that the practical, empirically evident limitations of security-in-use seem to indicate that, at this historical juncture, emancipatory political strategies not contingent on the successful redefinition of *security* as emancipation seem both more feasible and less dangerous.

From a different theoretical stance, while recognizing the dangers and risks associated with securitization, Elbe (2006) cautions against too readily seeking desecuritization, which he equates with the "politics as usual" that produced a devastatingly underwhelming response to HIV (Elbe, 2009). He suggests that the dangers associated with securitization could be mitigated by approaching HIV as security *issue*, not a security *threat*, and appealing to a "wider humanitarian framework ... compatible with a broadly Foucauldian perspective" (Elbe, 2009, p. 172). But if securitization requires threat construction and response (and Elbe, 2006) also seems to agree that this is the case), such an approach, while compatible with Foucault's typologies of power, is not compatible with the logic of securitization. And if, as I have argued, security-in-use in the UN system is so readily folded back into precisely this logic, it is not clear that security can realistically be invoked in the UN context (whether as a national or human security problem) without concomitant invocation of threat.

Hansen (2012) and MacKenzie (2010) share Elbe's concerns that desecuritization can result in inadequate political responses. They caution that desecuritization can produce silencing and exclusion, as in MacKenzie's study of female combatants in Sierra Leone who have been desecuritized through the international community's retroactive construction of their wartime identities as victims, not as (male) armed combatants. While combatants' return to civilian life is securitized as an urgent matter required to ensure peace, women as noncombatant 'victims' are, through desecuritization, excluded from post-conflict DDR programmes. "As a consequence, desecuritization is constituted as normatively and politically problematic" (Hansen, 2012, p. 544) in this analysis. Similarly the CS warns against "liberal desecuritization" (Buzan et al., 1998) that restricts securitization to the security sector while simultaneously desecuritizing other sectors, including the economic sector, in ways that legitimate exploitative economic relations between core and periphery states. While this mode of liberal desecuritization was perhaps more evident prior to 2001 and the re-securitization of global politics across sectors through the 'global war on terror', the broader point that desecuritization can too easily slide into support for a deeply unjust status quo is well-taken. However, at its core this is a critique of liberalism and the particular mode of desecuritization that it tends to produce; likewise, Hansen, MacKenzie and Elbe's critiques are all ultimately levelled at normal politics, which is equated with desecuritization in their analyses. This suggests not that we need to avoid desecuritization entirely, but that we need to avoid desecuritization strategies that are simply a return to apathy, complacency and depoliticization.

The significant accomplishments of global HIV activism suggest that alternatives beyond securitization exist and can effectively catalyse resource reallocation and "market transformations" (Kapstein & Busby, 2013). Yet these accomplishments, as Ingram (2013) points out, have been contingent and incomplete, and were largely achieved through the politics and rhetoric of exception, which may itself have been a strategy with ambiguous long-term consequences.[5] The gains made by positioning HIV as exceptional are, he argues, now at risk as the global response is folded back into neoliberal discourses of scarcity. If neither securitization nor broader claims of exceptionalism seem to have as much traction as they once did, we may now have reached a political moment in which strategies relying on exceptionalism, including but not limited to the strategies of securitization, are no longer likely to attract the attention of policymakers, or to successfully draw resources to the global HIV response. There may be no alternative to locating strategies in the terrain of desecuritized or normal politics.

This still leaves the question of why we ought to pursue desecuritization, rather than seeking an entirely different theoretical and political starting point. The answer is straightforward: empirically, HIV has been securitized, and it remains at least partially captured within the logic of threat construction and response, and the resulting exceptional practices, that characterize securitization. This is certainly the case in the UN's security response to HIV, and is arguably also the case in other facets of the global response (such as the criminalization of HIV transmission and other forms of HIV-related stigma). Having been securitized, any efforts to lift HIV out of security problematiques must necessarily begin with some form of desecuritization. That is, desecuritization is a necessary first step towards resituating an issue in the realm of normal politics.

I have also cautioned that there are continuities running between securitized and desecuritized politics, and that desecuritization is not sufficient to ensure the end or undoing of exceptional practices that settle, over time, into bureaucratic structures, practices and programmes. Therefore, the questions of desecuritization how, and into what, become especially important. If it entails, as Elbe, Hansen, MacKenzie, and the CS suggest it might, merely a return to pre-securitization complacency, desecuritization will simply perpetuate the inequities that have driven the global HIV pandemic, while leaving intact the existing exceptional practices of the security response to HIV, including displacement and deferral of human rights, ethically troubling HIV testing, and failure to provide ARV treatment.

Approaches to desecuritization

Eschewing securitization (or any politics of exception) need not mean accepting the status quo: we are not faced with the false choice of either securitization or politics as usual. Neither must desecuritization imply closure and return to an existing order. Desecuritization can entail not a capitulation and return to 'normal' in the sense of 'the way things were', but rather an approach that takes normal politics itself as both the site for and object of an agonistic, ongoing social justice project. Securitization, and exceptionalism more generally, can only ever catapult a single issue to the top of an existing political hierarchy, while leaving the hierarchy itself intact. By definition, exceptional practices occur outside of, and can therefore never transform, 'the normal' – and it is precisely the everyday practices of discrimination, stigma, racism, homophobia, gender-based violence, and myriad other forms of social exclusion that need to be confronted if we are to meaningfully address the structural drivers of HIV. What then, might such a project entail, and how can securitization theory be of any use?

While I have argued that securitization is limited as a social justice strategy, this does not mean that securitization *theory* cannot support normative and critical theorizing oriented towards social justice projects, including theorizing focused on desecuritization. Hansen (2012), reviewing extant theoretical and applied approaches to desecuritization, proposes a preliminary typology of four ideal types of desecuritization, each entailing, she argues, a different type of politics. While some of these forms are theorized as entailing a return to 'politics as usual', at least one holds the possibility of making normal politics the site and object of emancipatory struggle or resistance. Hansen hypothesizes that desecuritization can occur through: (1) stabilization, as in the case of Cold War détente; (2) replacement, in which "one issue [moves] out of security while another is simultaneously securitised" (541); (3) silencing, when an issue is unresolved but excluded from security discourse; and (4) rearticulation, wherein issues are desecuritized "by actively offering a political solution to the threats, dangers and grievances in question" (542). This typology is a useful starting point to consider how HIV has been, and might be, desecuritized without abandoning an emancipatory project.

To the extent that HIV has been desecuritized to date (notwithstanding that the ASCI report and Resolution 1983 represented an attempt to keep HIV securitized, and have been partly successful in that regard), the form this comes closest to in Hansen's typology is replacement. That is, the programmatic response has now partly settled into desecuritized bureaucratic structures, while other issues, notably the 'global war on terror', have assumed a more prominent place on the UNSC agenda and in the public imagination; even within the realm of global health, pandemic influenza (Rushton, 2011), other rapid-onset, high-mortality infectious diseases such as Ebola, and anti-microbial resistance are increasingly more likely than HIV to be the focus of global health security initiatives. Additionally, the changing meaning of 'HIV is a security threat' has now brought some populations and issues closer to the security response (women and girls, sexual violence as threat) while rendering others, central to the initial response, more marginal (peacekeepers as threat, the erasure of Africa). This replaces one set of threats and referent objects with another, constituting a form of replacement within HIV securitization.

If, as I have suggested, it is HIV's structural drivers that must be addressed, and if this would require undoing the threat-based logic of us/Other binaries, hierarchies and processes of exclusion – in short, if what is required is the transformation of normal politics itself – the form of desecuritization that holds greatest potential for this political project is rearticulation. Hansen (2012, p. 543) suggests that this can entail "fundamental transformations of the public sphere including a move out of the friend-enemy distinction... and of the identity and interests of Selves and Others"; yet she also cautions that this move "claims a finality, yet finality is inherently impossible" and wonders if rearticulation is "more akin to silencing than a genuine resolution" (p. 544).

But this is only one reading of what rearticulation could entail. Aradau's (2004) approach,[6] for example, recommends the invocation of rights, with a focus on "a gap or contradiction between these official principles and the actual practice – which excludes, by making them dangerous, pathological, abnormal, other groups" (p. 403). She elaborates that "[b]y virtue of their being [in principle] universally applicable, such rights can be reclaimed.... Those who are insecure can challenge the logic of security by claiming rights that are universally bestowed, but not applicable in practice to a specific category" (p. 404). This is not proposed as a naïve or simple solution: the terrain of struggle is shifted from the security to the legal field, and thus somewhat closer to normal politics, but this is the beginning of a political struggle and there is no implied finality or end. This is another point at which it is useful to think of desecuritization as existing on a Möbius strip, and to think of it as located within a policy and political process; this conception avoids finality, treating desecuritization, too, as a dynamic process characterized by ongoing interpretation and meaning-making contests.

This analysis may provide a conceptual or theoretical starting point, but what concretely does it suggest for desecuritizing HIV, achieving universal HIV treatment access, or advancing other social justice agendas? Renewed attention to the question of rights (including the right to health and protection from persecution on the basis of gender, racialization and sexual orientation) presents its own problems: law can and does exclude. It has been used by states to criminalize HIV transmission, restrict the cross-border travel of people living with HIV, and to persecute members of populations vulnerable to HIV including sex workers, MSM and people who use drugs. The right to health remains a contested concept (Davies, 2010), as do the broader social and economic rights of which the right to health is a subset (Evans, 2003). Furthermore, although centring the rights claims made by affected populations can privilege the voices and agency of some people living with and affected by HIV, processes of silencing, marginalization and the exercise of power are still very evident in struggles over who is authorized to speak for PHAs. It would be facile to suggest that rights claims expressed by social movements present 'the' solution to addressing HIV's structural drivers and creating a politics of solidarity.

Nevertheless, reaffirming that people living with, vulnerable to and affected by HIV are rights-bearers with positive claim *to* health, medicines, public goods, justice and full membership in a political community is one potential strategy for counteracting some of the problematic effects of the UNSC's HIV securitization (e.g. the displacement and deferral of human rights, and promotion of HIV testing without parallel commitment to provision of HIV treatment). It can also draw attention to the enduring limitations in the larger global response to HIV, including the failure to achieve universal treatment access, or, as discussed in Chapter 5, the failure to ensure that PEP is available to all women who have experienced sexual violence in the context of humanitarian emergencies. Rights language can convey moral urgency and outrage while also holding, even if this is sometimes more potential than actual, the legal force to compel changes in public goods provision. Especially when paired with the structural violence analyses that underpin most claims for social and economic rights (Farmer, 2001, 2003), it also holds the potential to catalyse longer-term structural change. Indeed, what structural change there has been to date in the provision of ARVs has been largely accomplished through the conjunction of social movement mobilization (Kapstein & Busby, 2013) and legal activism (Forman, 2013).

Legal claims contrasting the gap between universal principles and their uneven application in practice also have the effect of making normal politics itself the object of immanent critique by drawing attention to the failure of extant rights regimes and structures of public goods provision, as well as the political economies that have contributed to these failures. Drawing renewed attention to inequities in who can and cannot access ARVs and ethical HIV testing and support services identifies faults and failures in normal politics writ large, in the systems that privilege some lives over others and make this seem acceptable. It is an analysis from "a critical vantage point that requires thinking of our shared humanity less in terms of difference than inequality … [in which] we must think of the Other as self" (Fassin, 2007, p. xv). Such claims also, therefore, draw attention to the voices and experiences of the people who are ultimately most affected by HIV, most of whom are located in the global South and particularly in sub-Saharan Africa, and most of whom have all along been making claims rooted in rights and social justice, not security, language.

That we should attend to the rights of people living with and vulnerable to HIV is of course not a novel claim; this has been central to AIDS activism since the earliest days of the epidemic. My point is that, as I have argued elsewhere in this book, within the 'security response to HIV' that followed from the UNSC's resolutions and resulting programming, human rights have been displaced and deferred, and the people and places most affected by HIV have become increasingly less visible. Therefore, rights-based approaches offer one (though certainly not the only) strategy through which we might challenge international HIV securitization as it has actually been implemented and instantiated in programming and practice within the security response, and through which we might begin to undo the larger supporting logic of exclusion, threat construction and response, and us/Other binaries and hierarchies that have undergirded this response. I propose renewed attention to rights not as a panacea or magical solution to all the challenges faced by all the actors involved in the global response to HIV, but as one strategy, in one specific location, through which we might begin to pursue one component of a much larger social justice project.

Using the policy process framework to support desecuritization

Security studies and theories are not, as I have already acknowledged, the only theoretical vantage point from which to propose pathways out from or beyond securitization. But the securitization as policy process framework presented in this book offers one framework for structured analysis to identify opportunities for disrupting, resisting or challenging securitizations as they are underway, and for pursuing desecuritization of matters that have already been securitized. The primary aim of this book is to examine the origins and outcomes of the UNSC's HIV securitization, which has been underway for well over a decade at the time of writing. Therefore, the preceding chapters have used the securitization as policy process model to describe what empirically happened as HIV was securitized. This has entailed, for the most part, a descriptive analysis of what was and is, not a prescriptive discussion of what might have been or what could be. This analysis itself has utility for social justice praxis, since application of this framework can show exactly how and why securitization works, in practice, and how and why it is limited as a social justice strategy. It offers a negative lesson, in that it suggests what to avoid rather than what political strategies to pursue, but it is nevertheless useful given the continued allure of security and securitization – and the persistent perception on the part of both analysts and practitioners that securitization is a desirable and effective political strategy.

Beyond providing an analytical framework to study the emergence and effects of securitization, the securitization as policy process framework could equally be used to support a critical desecuritization project aimed at disrupting or resisting securitizing moves, or modes of rearticulation intended to move an issue into normal politics (which does not mean returning to the status quo, but rather entering a realm of contestation and resistance that is not bound by the exclusionary logic of securitization). If one were studying a securitization not in retrospect but as it unfolded, each stage of the policy process model could direct us toward interventions to undo, unmake or disrupt securitization.

In studying the speech act and the historical conditions of its emergence, we can ask, what are the opportunities to resist, remake or reframe threat constructions? Given that contests, at this stage, are likely to take place primarily at the level of discourse and primarily among elites, what counter-hegemonic discourses could be mobilized in response, and at whom should these be directed? At the framing contest stage, which is also mainly discursive and mainly among elite securitizing actors, critical analysis can identify and mobilize alternate frames that might disrupt the binaries of threatened and threatening subjects. Both of these stages, in other words, present opportunities for the type of rearticulation proposed by Hansen (2012) or the "process of dis-identification" recommended by Aradau (2004).

The policy implementation stage, which includes boundary work undertaken as securitizing directives are interpreted by bureaucratic actors, as well as the programme development and delivery undertaken by frontline staff, provides further opportunities to challenge and disrupt securitization, including efforts to undo us/Other boundaries by drawing attention to the gap between principles (such as human rights) and the exclusionary practices of securitization. Finally, the policy learning stage, especially in cases where there are dense interconnections between actors and analysts, offers the opportunity to articulate alternate approaches that might return an issue to normal politics, and to clearly demonstrate the problematic effects of securitization.

To reiterate, this is not proffered as a blanket prescription or blueprint for action in the entire global response to HIV, or any other social justice struggle. Those pursuing social justice objectives relating to issues that have never been securitized, or working in areas of the global HIV response that are not primarily unfolding within the threat-based logic of securitization, have a diverse array of political strategies at their disposal.[7] But to the extent that issues, once securitized, are captured within this cycle, the securitization as policy process framework can help us identify where, how, and through engagement with whom we might disrupt securitizing practices and logics, thereby beginning desecuritization processes that would enable a return to (agonistic, contested) normal politics.

Conclusion

The international securitization of HIV in and through the UNSC has produced at once limited and problematic results. This chapter has argued that these limitations and problems are inherent to the logic of securitization itself, though they were also exacerbated by the organizational context of the UN system which, with its deeply institutionalized understandings of what security 'really means', has produced a form of security-in-use that is largely equated and conflated with the security sector, militaries, and national security problematiques. Consequently, HIV's structural drivers cannot be addressed within a securitized response, which is predicated on maintaining the very binaries, boundaries and hierarchies between us and Other that enabled the pandemic to take hold, and that have worked to make the people and places most affected by and vulnerable to HIV also least able to access ARVs. In light of these limitations, I have suggested that desecuritization strategies, undertaken with the aim of making normal politics the site of emancipatory praxis, are warranted. Such strategies might include, though they are by no means limited to, rights-based rearticulation within the security response, and use of the securitization as policy process framework to identify opportunities to disrupt and unmake the threat-based logic, discourse and practices of securitization.

This should not be read as a foreclosure or abandonment of emancipatory and critical possibilities; the analysis simply takes actually-existing securitization dynamics, processes and practices as the starting point for pursuit of these possibilities. Normative analysis in and through securitization theory, including through use of the securitization as policy process framework presented in this book, is quite compatible with and capable of supporting a Coxian critical project which

> allows for a normative choice in favour of a social and political order different from the prevailing order, but ... limits the range of choices to alternative orders which are feasible transformations of the existing world. A principal objective of critical theory, therefore, is to clarify this range of possible alternatives ... it can represent a coherent picture of an alternative order, but ... [i]t must reject improbable alternatives just as it rejects the permanency of the existing order.
>
> (Cox, 1981, p. 130)

While in principle the dominant meanings of security-in-use that facilitated HIV securitization could change, in actually existing international relations practice, and certainly in the UN system, 'security' has a dominant and deeply entrenched meaning. The logic of securitization is similarly predicated on deeply entrenched threat discourses and assumptions about what and who is "generally held to be threatening" (Buzan et al., 1998, p. 33). These work together to produce the actually existing conditions in which securitizations are undertaken and security is spoken. It is then essential to a critical or any broadly normative project that we seek "feasible transformations of the existing world" by engaging with and seeking to disrupt and undo actually existing securitizations, including through desecuritization strategies as outlined, albeit in a preliminary manner, in this chapter.

Notes

1 Treatment as prevention approaches, for example, recommend the initiation of treatment as soon as possible after diagnosis, with the aim of achieving an undetectable viral load (which greatly reduces risk of HIV transmission) in the newly diagnosed patient; these approaches also, therefore, recommend greatly scaled-up and routinized HIV testing. While this is of course undertaken in part to promote the health of PHAs, it also, by emphasizing prevention as the ultimate goal, constitutes a form of intervention into PHA bodies in order to defend and protect HIV-negative people against those bodies. It may constitute the emergence of a "new biomedical norm", requiring mobilization of disciplinary and biopower, similar to that identified by Elbe (2009, p. 19).
2 WHO eligibility guidelines for HIV treatment have since changed. With new guidelines now recommending initiation of treatment as soon as possible after diagnosis, regardless of viral load, the number of people eligible for treatment but not receiving it has now increased (World Health Organization (WHO), 2015). Thus, in spite of the congratulatory rhetoric of the UNAIDS "15 by 15" report, which describes the goal of 15 million people receiving ARV treatment by 2015 as "a target achieved" (Joint United Nations Programme on HIV/AIDS (UNAIDS), 2015) we are still far short of the goal of universal, or even equitable, treatment access.

3 For a similar critique of the inability of securitization to address structural drivers, especially gendered vulnerability, see Seckinelgin et al. (2010).
4 For a useful critique of emancipation as it is conceived in some security-as-emancipation literature, see Peoples (2011).
5 Huysmans (2008), though from a different theoretical vantage point, is similarly critical of the "jargon of exception" and the politics it produces (and forecloses).
6 Hansen suggests that Aradau's project is a form of change through stabilization; yet my reading of Aradau's call for using rights as a means of "establishing a political link with the other" (Aradau, 2004, p. 405) suggests an attempt to move out of us/Other or friend-enemy distinctions – which seems closer to Hansen's ideal type of rearticulation.
7 However, because policy processes are not unique to securitization, policy process models could also be used to identify opportunities for social justice intervention in 'normal politics' policy development and implementation.

References

Aradau, Claudia. (2004). Security and the democratic scene: desecuritization and emancipation. *Journal of International Relations and Development*, *7*(4), 388–413.
Balzacq, Thierry. (2011). A theory of securitization: origins, core assumptions, variants. In Thierry Balzacq (Ed.), *Securitization Theory: How Security Problems Emerge and Dissolve* (pp. 1–30). New York: Routledge.
Balzacq, Thierry (Ed.). (2015). *Contesting Security: Strategies and Logics*. New York: Routledge.
Barnett, Tony & Whiteside, Alan. (2006). *AIDS in the Twenty-First Century: Disease and Globalization* (2nd ed.). New York: Palgrave Macmillan.
Basu, Soumita. (2011). Security as emancipation: a feminist perspective. In J. Ann Tickner & Laura Sjoberg (Eds.), *Feminism and International Relations: Conversations about the past, present and future* (pp. 98–114). Abingdon: Routledge.
Bigo, Didier. (2005). La mondialisation de l'(in)sécurité?: Réflexions sur le champ des professionnels de la gestion des inquiétudes et analytique de la transnationalisation des processus d'(in)sécurisation. *Cultures & Conflits*, *58*(2), 53–101.
Booth, Ken. (1991). Security and emancipation. *Review of International Studies*, *17*(4), 313–326.
Booth, Ken. (2005). Beyond critical security studies. In Ken Booth (Ed.), *Critical Security Studies in World Politics* (pp. 259–278). Boulder, CO: Lynne Rienner.
Browning, Christopher S. & McDonald, Matt. (2011). The future of critical security studies: ethics and the politics of security. *European Journal of International Relations*, *19*(2), 235–255.
Buzan, Barry, Wæver, Ole, & de Wilde, Jaap. (1998). *Security: A New Framework for Analysis*. Boulder, CO: Lynne Rienner.
Cox, Robert W. (1981). Social forces, states and world orders: beyond international relations theory. *Millennium*, *10*(2), 126–155.
Davies, Sara E. (2010). What contribution can international relations make to the evolving global health agenda? *International Affairs*, *86*(5), 1167–1190.
Elbe, Stefan. (2006). Should HIV/AIDS be securitized? The ethical dilemma of linking HIV/AIDS and security. *International Studies Quarterly*, *50*(1), 199–144.
Elbe, Stefan. (2009). *Virus Alert: Security, Governmentality, and the AIDS Pandemic*. New York: Columbia University Press.
Evans, Tony. (2003). A human right to health? *Third World Quarterly*, *23*(2), 197–215.

Farmer, Paul. (2001). *Infections and Inequalities: The Modern Plagues.* Berkeley, CA: University of California Press.

Farmer, Paul. (2003). *Pathologies of Power: Health, Human Rights and the New War on the Poor.* Berkeley, CA: University of California Press.

Fassin, Didier. (2007). *When Bodies Remember: Experiences and Politics of AIDS in South Africa* (Amy Jacobs & Gabrielle Varro, Trans.). Berkeley, CA: University of California Press.

Floyd, Rita. (2007). Towards a consequentialist evaluation of security: bringing together the Copenhagen and the Welsh Schools of security studies. *Review of International Studies*, (33), 327–350.

Floyd, Rita. (2011). Can securitization theory be used in normative analysis? Towards a just securitization theory. *Security Dialogue*, *42*(4–5), 427–439.

Forman, Lisa. (2013). What contribution have human rights approaches made to reducing AIDS-related vulnerability in sub-Saharan Africa? Exploring the case study of access to antiretrovirals. *Global Health Promotion*, *20*(Supp. 1), 57–63.

Hansen, Lene. (2012). Reconstructing desecuritization: the normative-political in the Copenhagen School and directions for how to apply it. *Review of International Studies*, *38*, 525–546.

Hunter, Mark. (2010). *Love in the Time of AIDS: Inequality, Gender and Rights in South Africa.* Bloomington, IN: Indiana University Press.

Huysmans, Jef. (2008). The jargon of exception – on Schmitt, Agamben and the absence of political society. *International Political Sociology*, *2*, 165–183.

Ingram, Alan. (2013). After the exception: HIV/AIDS beyond salvation and scarcity. *Antipode*, *45*(2), 436–454.

Joint United Nations Programme on HIV/AIDS (UNAIDS). (2013). Access to antiretro-viral therapy in Africa: status report on progress towards the 2015 targets Retrieved 18 January 2016 from www.unaids.org/sites/default/files/media_asset/20131219_AccessARTAfricaStatusReportProgresstowards2015Targets_en_0.pdf.

Joint United Nations Programme on HIV/AIDS (UNAIDS). (2014). The Gap Report. Retrieved 20 January 2016 from www.unaids.org/en/resources/documents/2014.

Joint United Nations Programme on HIV/AIDS (UNAIDS). (2015). "15 by 15": a global target achieved. Retrieved 18 January 2016 from www.unaids.org/en/resources/documents/2015/15_by_15_a_global_target_achieved.

Kapstein, Ethan B. & Busby, Joshua W. (2013). *AIDS Drugs for All: Social Movements and Market Transformations.* Cambridge, UK: Cambridge University Press.

MacKenzie, Megan. (2010). Securitization and de-securitization: female soldiers and the reconstruction of women in post-conflict Sierra Leone. In Laura Sjoberg (Ed.), *Gender and International Security: Feminist Perspectives* (pp. 151–167). New York: Routledge.

Mugyenyi, Peter. (2008). *Genocide By Denial: How Profiteering From HIV/AIDS Killed Millions.* Kampala: Fountain Publishers.

Nguyen, Vinh-Kim. (2010). *The Republic of Therapy: Triage and Sovereignty in West Africa's Time of AIDS.* Durham, NC: Duke University Press.

Nunes, João. (2012). Reclaiming the political: emancipation and critique in security studies. *Security Dialogue*, *43*(4), 345–361.

Nunes, João. (2014). *Security, Emancipation and the Politics of Health: A New Theoretical Perspective.* New York: Routledge.

O'Byrne, Patrick, Bryan, Alyssa, & Roy, Marie (2013). HIV Criminal Prosecutions and Public Health: An Examination of the Empirical Research. *BMJ Medical Humanities*, *39*(2), 85–90.

Patton, Cindy. (1990). *Inventing AIDS*. New York: Routledge.

Peoples, Columba. (2011). Security after emancipation? Critical theory, violence and resistance. *Review of International Studies, 37*(3), 1113–1135.

Piot, Peter. (2006). AIDS: from crisis management to sustained strategic response. *The Lancet, 368*(9534), 526–530.

Roe, Paul. (2012). Is securitization a "negative" concept? Revisiting the normative debate over normal versus extraordinary politics. *Security Dialogue, 43*(3), 249–266.

Rushton, Simon. (2010). AIDS and international security in the United Nations system. *Health Policy and Planning, 25*, 495–504.

Rushton, Simon. (2011). Global health security: security for whom? Security from what? *Political Studies, 59*(4), 779–796.

Salter, Mark B. (2008). Securitization and desecuritization: a dramaturgical analysis of the Canadian Air Transport Security Authority. *Journal of International Relations and Development, 11*(4), 321–349.

Seckinelgin, Hakan, Bigirumwami, Joseph, & Morris, Jill. (2010). Securitization of HIV/ AIDS in context: gendered vulnerability in Burundi. *Security Dialogue, 41*(5), 515–535.

Whiteside, Alan & Smith, Julia. (2009). Exceptional epidemics: AIDS still deserves a global response. *Globalization and Health, 5*(15). doi: 10.1186/1744–8603–5-15

World Health Organization (WHO). (2015). Treat all people living with HIV, offer antiretrovirals as additional prevention choice for people at "substantial" risk. Retrieved 18 January 2016 from www.who.int/mediacentre/news/releases/2015/hiv-treat-all-recommendation/en/.

8 Conclusion

This book has undertaken three inter-related inquiries. First was the empirical evaluation of HIV securitization in the UN system, intended to assess the extent to which securitizing strategies are effective at supporting social justice projects by drawing attention and resources to an issue and catalysing transformation in how and to whom those resources are distributed. This also served as a means of testing the beliefs, widely held by actors in international politics and many IR theorists, that the invocation of security holds special political power and that securitization is an effective if often illiberal problem-solving strategy. Second, analytically and theoretically, the book sought to advance securitization theory (especially its empirical application and use) by reimagining securitization as a policy process. This framework knits together Copenhagen and sociological variants of securitization theory into a single analytical model; by encompassing discourses, speech acts, bureaucratic practices and programmes, and multiple levels of actors and analysis, it provides a systematic, structured means of studying 'real world' securitizations from origins to outcomes. It additionally, as suggested in Chapter 7, can support normative and critical desecuritization projects by identifying opportunities to resist, revise or undo securitizations as they unfold. The application of this model to the empirical case of international HIV securitization then supported the book's third aim: a normative assessment of the ethics and efficacy of securitization as a social justice strategy.

The argument has been that securitization relies on the invocation of threat, which produces us/Other hierarchies and a narrow, oppositional politics of threat response predicated on defence against the Other. It is therefore inherently limited as a means to social justice ends, and this is especially so in contexts, including the UN system (and arguably the larger contemporary context of the global war on terror), where security-in-use is already largely defined in national security terms and conflated with the security sector. But the book has also shown that international HIV securitization has been less static than often assumed. It has evolved significantly over time, inverting and reversing the original arguments about how and to whom HIV is a security threat, such that even as the logic of securitization was a constant constraint, the referent objects and assumed source of the threat in 2011 were quite different than they were in 2000. This inversion and evolution was catalysed, in large part, by interactions between securitizing actors and analysts, who learned from each other and worked together to produce security knowledge.

The analysis illustrates that securitizations need to be studied as dynamic, evolving, ongoing meaning-making contests, and that the securitization as policy process framework, which supports contextualized, historical analysis that foregrounds contestation and change, is especially useful in this regard. It also illustrates that securitization theory is inherently political. We as analysts cannot claim some analytical vantage point comfortably above or outside of security politics. As such, the ethical and normative dimensions of our work matter deeply: it has the potential to influence not just IR but security actors, practices and politics, though of course this potential will vary by context and by issue. Further development of desecuritization as a concept and political strategy (including the preliminary discussion in Chapter 7 about how the securitization as policy process model might be of use in this endeavour) therefore continues to be among the most important of the ongoing intellectual and political projects in securitization theory and the broader field of security studies. This will also require sustained engagement with theories and fields beyond security studies.

By way of conclusion, then, this chapter summarizes the contributions the book makes to this larger project, as well as the avenues for future research that it has opened. I begin with a brief discussion of the utility of the policy process model and of careful attention to security-in-use in empirical studies of securitization, and then turn to two recurring themes in the book that suggest the need for further engagement with literature and traditions beyond security studies: these are the simultaneous presence and absence of Africa in international HIV securitization, and the relationship between securitization, desecuritization and social change.

This chapter focuses mainly on what the book contributes to security studies, not what it contributes to the global response to HIV (or to the global health literature that studies that response). This is not because the latter consideration is unimportant, or because the book has little to offer the global response. On the contrary, my primary impetus when I began this project was to understand the impact of securitization on the global response and people living with HIV in order to consider how and in what ways this global response, still incomplete and only partially successful, could be made not only more effective but more just. The contribution the book makes to this and other social justice projects – the substantial new empirical detail about HIV securitization, the warning that securitization as a social justice strategy is both dangerous and of limited effectiveness, and the recommendation that we pursue desecuritization strategies that make normal politics the focus of emancipatory praxis – has however been clearly conveyed in the previous chapters. By outlining the book's contributions to security studies, we can now uncover several further research inquiries, some of which could also be of use in future research oriented specifically towards HIV securitization and the politics of the global response.

Securitization as a policy process, revisited

The book has shown, including through empirical application, that a policy process framework can productively resolve some of the tensions between CS and sociological variants of securitization theory; it can support the structured, systematic empirical investigation of securitization in ways that appropriately consider history and context; and it can support normative and critical studies of securitization's effects. Approaching securitization as a policy process additionally provides us with different and productive ways to think about scale, levels of analysis and authority in securitization.

Linking scales and levels of analysis

As discussed in Chapter 4, HIV securitization entailed interactions between 'local' and 'global' actors: the carefully curated encounters with AIDS orphans and women living with HIV that UNAIDS arranged for Richard Holbrooke in Namibia (Piot, 2009; Sternberg, 2002); Holbrooke's spontaneous, incidental witnessing of peacekeepers and sex workers in Cambodia (PBS, 2006); and Piot's extensive experience as a medical professional researching HIV in multiple African countries prior to the advent of ARVs (Piot, 2012). The local and global were linked through encounters and interactions between securitizing elites and the 'local' populations who then became both the impetus for and the ultimate objects of securitizing moves. In HIV securitization, actors working in the service of states, the UN and the international community, attempting to achieve securitization at the global or international level, were prompted to do so partly as a result of experiences at the level of the 'local' and 'everyday'. First-hand interactions served as the mechanism that linked local insecurity to an international-level securitizing move; it was the securitization process itself, not merely the issue (in this case HIV),[1] that traversed multiple scales. Methodologically, this indicates the need for careful empirical consideration of what Avant et al. (2010) call "the microfoundations of global politics" – the formal and informal networks and interpersonal connections that underpin global-level policymaking – which, as this book has shown, can occur across as well as within different levels.

These encounters also offer new ways to think about the relationship between 'the local' and 'the global'. Interactions between policy-makers and 'local' people may serve as an analytical bridge, allowing us to think about securitization and securitizing moves as occurring on several different levels simultaneously – or, in ways that may be both more productive and more problematic, of not thinking about local/national/global levels as separate and distinct, but rather as overlapping and interconnected. This complicates existing security studies engagements with scale, which have ranged from calls to refocus attention to the local "everyday human (in)security" at the level of cities (Lemanski, 2012), to the need for scaled-up analyses of "macrosecuritizations" occurring between middle-level and system-level securitizations (Buzan & Wæver, 2009), to the suggestion that securitizations can occur sequentially across scales, beginning at the domestic and then moving to the international in ways that may support macrosecuritizing moves (McInnes & Rushton, 2013).[2] All of these approach how and at what level securitization occurs as largely an either-or question: securitization is understood as originating at one level, though there may then be cause-effect relationships across levels. The securitization as policy process framework opens up consideration of how levels from local to global are connected and interlinked through securitization processes, and of how these connections and linkages might be studied empirically.

It additionally opens up new approaches to thinking about securitizing actors and audiences. While it has not been a focus of analysis in this book, approaching securitization as a policy process in which actors move from 'local' (community-based programmes or peacekeeping missions) to 'global' policy spheres (the UNSC or UNAIDS offices in Geneva), and in which securitizations unfold in multiple locations (high-level sessions at the UNSC, multiple offices across the UN system, and UN peace missions), can help us explore in a structured manner how actors' identities shift depending upon their location. Holbrooke was a securitizing actor in the UNSC, but he was also the audience for the security claims of Namibian women living with HIV; UNSC member state delegates were simultaneously actors and audience as they debated the meaning of 'HIV is a security threat'; and the mid-level bureaucratic actors tasked with implementing Resolution 1308 were one of the audiences for the resolution, but they themselves became securitizing actors as they developed programmes to address the sexual behaviour of peacekeepers. The identities of securitizing actors and audiences in this case are dynamic and multiple. This shows that the categories of 'audience' and 'actor' can overlap, and people may play both roles, either sequentially or simultaneously, at different stages of the policy process. This framework then opens up new and potentially very fruitful approaches to theorizing 'the audience', a central concern of sociological approaches to securitization (Balzacq, 2005; Léonard & Kaunert, 2011; Salter, 2008; Williams, 2011).

The securitizing authority of non-state actors

In addition to opening up new ways of thinking about actors and audiences, the framework also shows how securitizing authority can be exercised by non-state actors. This presents new opportunities to theorize how authority is exercised, both in and beyond securitizations, and to engage with a rich constructivist global governance literature.

The question of who, empirically, has the authority to securitize is left open in the CS framework; while the securitizing actor must be "in a position of authority", "this should not be defined as official authority" (Buzan, Wæver, & de Wilde, 1998, p. 33). However, because the original framework is (1) mainly focused on the "middle level" of states (Buzan & Wæver, 2009), and (2) has a high (though not entirely clearly established) threshold for exceptionalism and rule-breaking (Williams, 2011), authority in securitization has often been seen to be held by states. Buzan and Waever's (2009) discussion of macrosecuritizations does create greater empirical and theoretical room for the exercise of securitizing authority by transnational actors, while Hameiri and Jones (2012) suggest that non-traditional security threats entailing securitization above the national level can implicate non-state as well as state actors. Still, securitization theory, especially in its more Schmittian forms, has been criticized for being too state-centric, and therefore unable to recognize forms of authority exercised by non-state actors, especially in the global South (Barthwal-Datta, 2009).

The policy process model usefully addresses this critique and builds on existing attempts to theorize non-state actors as securitizing agents, as it shows that the exercise of authority (both who can exercise it, and what forms it can take) can, first, vary depending on the stage of the policy process. While the speech act marks one visible moment of decision, in which authority is exercised mainly by elite actors (in this case, the UNSC, especially the P5, and executive-level UN staff), bureaucratic actors and frontline staff are also able to influence how high-level securitizing directives are interpreted and implemented. Meaning-making contests and political struggles are ongoing, and authority can be exercised by diverse actors at different stages of the policy process.

Second, by focusing on how securitizations unfold in a particular organizational or bureaucratic setting, the framework treats authority not as an absolute, Schmittian expression of sovereign power, but as context-dependent decision-making that includes the power to break rules *within a given structure or setting* (in this case, the UN system). Exception, that is, is not absolute; it is always contextual and relative, situated within particular policies and politics. As discussed in Chapter 2, policies can be enacted in response to perceived threats, and context-specific rules broken, in NGOs, neighbourhood groups, firms, and myriad other non-state actors. A policy process model therefore provides us with a framework to systematically examine the context in which securitizing authority is exercised, and to identify which actors have authority, of what form, in a given context. This in turn helps us to identify where to look (and what to look for) to identify the rule-breaking authority that characterizes securitization.

This creates potential for new conversations between securitization theory and constructivist global governance literature, which has similarly explored the question of what sort of power and authority non-state actors can exercise, under what conditions, in which specific organizational contexts (Avant, Finnemore, & Sell, 2010; Barnett & Finnemore, 2004; Willetts, 2011).[3] Barnett and Finnemore (2004), for example, identify the delegated, moral and expert authority of international organizations (IOs), while Avant et al. (2010) identify institutional, delegated, expert, principled and capacity-based forms of authority exercised by non-state global governance actors with multiple, overlapping spheres of influence. Future research could usefully explore how and in what ways these forms of authority can be parlayed into securitizing authority, or mobilized to challenge and resist securitizing authority (including resistance in support of desecuritization strategies of the sort discussed in Chapter 7). Investigating authority and/in securitization also requires much deeper engagement with postcolonial theory (Epstein, 2014), a point to which I return below.

Security-in-use: the relations between ideas, institutions and policy

The book has also focused on security-in-use: how 'security', as a word, concept and set of practices, was actually used and understood by actors implicated in HIV securitization and the resulting security response to HIV. This analytical focus stems from the recognition that while security is an essentially contested concept, it is contested precisely because many practitioners and academics alike in fact hold very strong views about what security 'really means'. Some analysts insist that security has an inherent negative logic (Aradau, 2004; Huysmans, 2006; Seckinelgin, 2012); security as emancipation theorists are equally certain that it does not (Booth, 2007, 2005; Nunes, 2014). Browning and McDonald (2011, p. 251) therefore call for contextualized analysis "of the ways in which security is constructed and challenged in particular social, historical and political contexts", which is precisely the analysis the securitization as policy process model is meant to support. I have already outlined in the introduction why careful attention to security, the word, is an important component of this analysis, and then demonstrated the empirical operations and impact of security-in-use in international HIV securitization. Tracing how 'security' is actually deployed can also support analysis of the relationship between ideas, institutions and policy outcomes.

A core argument of this book has been that through the securitization policy process, ideas, discourse, practices and learning interact to produce material consequences. Securitization is an iterative policy process: ideas (about threat, race, disease, security, and strategies for political action), emerge in and through discursive histories that shape who or what is 'thinkable' as a threat, and who falls into the categories of threatening and threatened. As ideas coalesce, that is, as securitizing actors interpret the material world through these discourses and determine courses of political action, they engage in securitizing speech that, articulated in specific policy and organizational contexts, then triggers meaning-making contests that eventually resolve into broadly though not universally shared understandings about policy problems and solutions. These then produce policy directives, programmes and practices that have material impact, influencing how and to whom goods such as HIV treatment are distributed.

This is not a deterministic process. At each stage of the policy process, meaning-making contests can shift the boundaries between threatening and threatened, replace one referent object with another, or revise the exact content of a threat response. However, throughout, deeply path-dependent and institutionalized meanings of security shape the parameters of what is recognized as securitizing speech and recognized as security practice, as well as which actors in a given context are understood as having the authority to act on security matters.

This affirms that ideas about security, to borrow Risse-Kappen's (1994) phrase, "do not float freely": they interact with and are manifested through structures, and it is this interaction that determines the exact contours of resulting policy directives, security practices, and bodily and territorial impacts. Put differently, securitization always takes place in a political and organizational context, and that context includes prior beliefs about what security 'really means', as well as organizational structures, divisions of authority and entrenched practices that reflect these prior definitions of security. Policy outcomes then need to be understood as the result of this dynamic, but constrained, interaction between ideas about security and the institutions in and through which security is spoken and practiced.

Africa and/in IR and security studies

A central argument of this book has been that we cannot make sense of HIV securitization without considering the role and use of Africa in this securitization. As discussed in Chapter 3, this securitization depended upon discursive linkages between HIV and Africa, both of which had already been constructed as threatening; furthermore, assertions about the devastating impact of HIV on Africans' security, health and well-being were the ostensible reason for the January 2000 UNSC session that first securitized HIV. Subsequent policy directives (Resolutions 1308 and 1983), however, did not address the African pandemic, although African states and peacekeepers continued to be invisibly but deeply implicated in resulting programmes and practices. Consequently, the southern African states and people who continue to be most affected by HIV, and to experience significant treatment access barriers (Joint United Nations Programme on HIV/AIDS (UNAIDS), 2013, 2014, 2015), were excluded from the UN's securitized response to HIV.

The gradual erasure of Africa, and the resulting silence at the core of the UNSC's HIV securitization, was mirrored in subsequent academic analysis of the UNSC sessions. Some analyses note in passing that HIV was securitized with reference to Africa, but the significant shift from HIV as a threat to security in Africa in the January 2000 UNSC sessions, to a threat to (and originating in) peacekeepers in Resolution 1308, to a threat somewhat nebulously associated with sexual violence in Resolution 1983, has not been problematized. Rather, the 'dropping out' of Africa from the conversation immediately following dire proclamations about the impact of HIV on the continent has largely gone unremarked,[4] perpetuating the present-but-invisible status of Africa that was empirically evident in the UNSC sessions and subsequent security response to HIV.

The book has sought to somewhat rectify this silence by examining how ideas about Africa were deployed in the service of HIV securitization, and how Africa and Africans were rendered less visible over time; this analysis has included reading the UNSC sessions and associated discussions through Mbembe (2001, 2003) to uncover how Africa is used as a signifier of disease, disorder and threat in the discourses that underpin HIV securitization. By placing the status of Africa in HIV securitization at the centre of analysis, examining what work the initial invocation of Africa did, for whom, as well as the material consequences this invocation did (and did not) produce, and by asking how we should make sense of the continent's shifting status and gradual erasure, the book is one contribution to a much larger project of addressing disciplinary silences and erasures in security studies and IR.

With some recent exceptions (Anievas, Manchanda, & Shilliam, 2015; Barkawi & Laffey, 2006; Bilgin, 2008; Brown, 2012; Dunn & Shaw, 2001; Epstein, 2014; Shilliam, 2010; M. Smith, 2005), many of which are part of a larger turn to 'decolonizing IR', Africa (and the global South more broadly) has rarely been central to IR theory-building and empirical research. In one response to this lacuna, Harman and Brown (2013, p. 86) critique a tendency in IR theory to draw upon "stereotypical images of Africa", arguing that in response Africa should be brought "in from the margins" of IR scholarship through use of African cases to critically examine IR theories, analytical concepts, and how North/South power relations structure IR knowledge production. To this I would add the importance of tracing how, when and why Africa is invoked in international relations, and conversely, when and why international actors are silent about Africa and the impact of policies and practices on African states and peoples: for the invocation of "stereotypical images of Africa" is endemic to international relations as well as to IR, and these images and ideas have material consequences. Thompson (2015, p. 45), following Stoler, further argues that IR is characterized by a "racial aphasia": a wilful forgetting of and collective silence about the racist foundations of contemporary IR and international politics.

These analyses all point to the need for security studies and securitization theory to engage far more deeply with critical race and postcolonial theory. Normative analysis in securitization theory, including investigations into the normative potential of desecuritization, provides one promising means in and through which to build dialogue between security studies and postcolonial theory. They share similar normative and political projects (though there are of course significant areas of disagreement); an interest in how power operates in and through discourse in ways that then have material effects; and an interest in uncovering how difference operates to construct self and Other. In addition to helping us think through the ways that securitizing authority can operate as an expression of racial power, postcolonial and critical race theory also offer theories and praxis for undoing (or at least making visible and troubling) us/Other boundaries and hierarchies. They are therefore an essential component of any effort to theorize and enact desecuritization projects.

De/securitization and social change

This brings us to the question of how to think about and enact social change; especially, what is the relationship between securitization, desecuritization and social change, and how might desecuritization be set in motion in ways that support social justice objectives? This book sought to carefully evaluate the efficacy of international HIV securitization as a means of achieving social justice ends, not to propose a blueprint for future action but to uncover lessons (especially about the limitations of securitization) to generally guide or inform efforts to trigger redistributive or transformative political action. As such, the question of exactly what desecuritization into normal politics, in a way that makes normal politics the site for social justice praxis, might entail, is not one that the book on its own can answer; it is raised here simply to identify an avenue for future research.

Consideration of these questions is also the point at which securitization theory needs to look beyond the borders of security studies to engage with other theories of social change, especially those of social movement literature – which, like engagement with postcolonial and critical race theory, could generate fruitful cross-disciplinary dialogue. In addition to Keck and Sikkink's (1998) well-known work on transnational advocacy and of course the many studies of HIV activism (e.g. Gray, 2012; Kapstein & Busby, 2013; Nunn et al., Smith & Siplon, 2006), an emerging literature that examines the tactics and forms of authority exercised by social justice activists and organizations (e.g. Carpenter, 2014; Hendrix & Wong, 2013) could be usefully placed into dialogue with studies asking how the "normative-political" (Hansen, 2012) potential of desecuritization might be activated. For readers seeking very concrete prescriptions for action, the applied social movement literature also provides practical activist strategies that securitization theory, as a theory, cannot and is not designed to provide.

Conclusion

HIV securitization, and the interventions such securitization authorizes or fails to achieve, is a political issue with profound human consequences. As one interviewee observed:

> At the end of the day, what it is about are the people on the ground. Do they have what they need in order to keep from contracting HIV? In the event that they do contract HIV, do they have what they need in order for them not to pass it on to somebody else? In order for them to live the quality of life that is possible given the advances of science in this era?... Are we asking ourselves, as actors in HIV, are we asking ourselves these questions every day? Because at the end of the day, there's a man, there's a woman, there's a child, there's a baby who is affected by what answers we give when these questions are asked.
>
> (Eric, 2010)

This book has suggested that "the people on the ground", those who are most affected by and vulnerable to HIV, have not significantly benefitted from the significant time, effort and money expended to place HIV on the UNSC agenda, nor from the resulting 'security response to HIV'. Furthermore, those who have been impacted by this security response – mainly UN peacekeepers – have been reached via ethically troubling HIV testing strategies, but not by similarly concerted efforts to provide HIV treatment. In the wider global response that securitization was intended to support, many of the people and places most affected by HIV are still, notwithstanding significant improvements in treatment distribution, unable to access ARVs.

Securitization did not and could not catalyse the structural changes that would be required to meaningfully address HIV; it is inherently constrained by a logic that produces exceptional but oppositional defensive response, predicated on hierarchies and binaries that sharply delineate between a threatened inside and a threatening outside. As a transformative strategy, securitization is therefore necessarily incomplete at best and unjust at worst. Addressing HIV and its structural drivers certainly requires concerted global response, but securitization cannot produce the type of response we require. Such a response would need to avoid both the constrained, threat-based logic of securitization and the deficiencies of normal politics; entail not breaking but changing the rules and norms that determine how resources are allocated and whose lives matter most; and produce not exceptions to but a fundamental transformation of normal politics itself. Neither securitization nor the terrible, quiet complicity of the status quo will get us there.

Notes

1 This is a different approach than the original CS stance that "[i]t is possible to mix levels and have, for example, local causes and global effects … or global causes and local effects….This situation, however, is all about the level of the *issue*, not necessarily of its securitization" (Buzan & Wæver, 2009, p. 17).
2 While McInnes and Rushton (2013) suggest that HIV securitization originated in US domestic politics and then cascaded internationally, the analysis in this book suggests that, first, there was a distinct international-level move to securitize HIV, undertaken by Piot and UNAIDS for reasons independent of US politics; and second, that the content and meaning of these securitizations were very different, such that when we compare international HIV securitization in 2000, in 2011, and in US military and intelligence circles in the 1990s, we are comparing three different and not fully compatible articulations of 'HIV is a security threat'.
3 An emerging global health governance literature (Davies, 2010; Fidler, 1997; Harman, 2012; McInnes & Lee, 2012), which is largely applied and empirical, could also be usefully developed through greater engagement with broader constructivist considerations of authority.
4 For an exception see O'Manique (2005). Elbe (2005, 2006) has also discussed the dangers of "biopolitical racism" directed at Africans, including in the context of securitization (though we have somewhat different definitions of securitization).

References

Anievas, Alexander, Manchanda, Nivi, & Shilliam, Robbie (Eds.). (2015). *Race and Racism in International Relations: Confronting the Global Colour Line*. New York: Routledge.

Aradau, Claudia. (2004). Security and the democratic scene: desecuritization and emancipation. *Journal of International Relations and Development*, 7(4), 388–413.

Avant, Deborah D., Finnemore, Martha, & Sell, Susan K. (Eds.). (2010). *Who Governs the Globe?* Cambridge, UK: Cambridge University Press.

Balzacq, Thierry. (2005). The three faces of securitization: political agency, audience and context. *European Journal of International Relations, 11*(2), 171–201.

Barkawi, Tarak & Laffey, Mark. (2006). The postcolonial moment in security studies. *Review of International Studies, 32*(2), 329–352.

Barnett, Michael & Finnemore, Martha. (2004). *Rules for the World: International Organizations in Global Politics.* Ithaca, NY: Cornell University Press.

Barthwal-Datta, Monika. (2009). Securitising threats without the state: a case study of misgovernance as a security threat in Bangladesh. *Review of International Studies, 35*(2), 277–300.

Bilgin, Pinar. (2008). Thinking past "Western" IR? *Third World Quarterly, 29*(1), 5–23.

Booth, Ken (Ed.). (2005). *Critical Security Studies in World Politics.* Boulder, CO: Lynne Rienner.

Booth, Ken. (2007). *Theory of World Security.* Cambridge, UK: Cambridge University Press.

Brown, William. (2012). A question of agency: Africa in international politics. *Third World Quarterly, 33*(10), 1889–1908

Browning, Christopher S. & McDonald, Matt. (2011). The future of critical security studies: Ethics and the politics of security. *European Journal of International Relations, 19*(2), 235–255.

Buzan, Barry & Wæver, Ole. (2009). Macrosecuritisation and security constellations: reconsidering scale in securitization theory. *Review of International Studies, 35*(2), 253–276.

Buzan, Barry, Wæver, Ole, & de Wilde, Jaap. (1998). *Security: A New Framework for Analysis.* Boulder, CO: Lynne Rienner.

Carpenter, Charli. (2014). *"Lost" Causes: Agenda Vetting in Global Issue Networks and the Shaping of Human Security.* Ithaca, NY: Cornell University Press.

Davies, Sara E. (2010). What contribution can international relations make to the evolving global health agenda? *International Affairs, 86*(5), 1167–1190.

Dunn, Kevin C. & Shaw, Timothy M. (Eds.). (2001). *Africa's Challenge to International Relations Theory.* New York: Palgrave.

Elbe, Stefan. (2005). AIDS, security, biopolitics. *International Relations, 19*(4), 403–419.

Elbe, Stefan. (2006). Should HIV/AIDS be securitized? The ethical dilemma of linking HIV/AIDS and security. *International Studies Quarterly, 50*(1), 199–144.

Epstein, Charlotte. (2014). The postcolonial perspective: an introduction. *International Theory, 6*(2), 294–311.

Eric (2010, 9 April). (Personal interview with author).

Fidler, David P. (1997). The globalization of public health: emerging infectious diseases and international relations. *Indiana Journal of Global Legal Studies, 5*(1), 11–51.

Gray, Dylan Mohan (Writer). (2012). *Fire in the blood.* In Dylan Mohan Gray (Producer). Ireland: Dartmouth Films & Films Transit.

Hameiri, Shahar & Jones, Lee. (2012). The politics and governance of non-traditional security. *International Studies Quarterly.* doi: 10.1111/isqu.12014

Hansen, Lene. (2012). Reconstructing desecuritization: the normative-political in the Copenhagen School and directions for how to apply it. *Review of International Studies, 38*, 525–546.

Harman, Sophie. (2012). *Global Health Governance.* New York: Routledge.

Harman, Sophie & Brown, William. (2013). In from the margins? The changing place of Africa in international relations. *International Affairs, 89*(1), 69–87.

Hendrix, Cullen S. & Wong, Wendy. (2013). Knowing your audience: how the structure of international relations and organizational choices affect Amnesty International's advocacy. *The Review of International Organizations, 9*(1), 29–58.

Huysmans, Jef. (2006). *The Politics of Insecurity: Fear, Migration and Asylum in the EU.* New York: Routledge.

Joint United Nations Programme on HIV/AIDS (UNAIDS). (2013). Access to antiretroviral therapy in Africa: status report on progress towards the 2015 targets Retrieved 18 January 2016 from www.unaids.org/sites/default/files/media_asset/20131219_AccessARTAfricaStatusReportProgresstowards2015Targets_en_0.pdf.

Joint United Nations Programme on HIV/AIDS (UNAIDS). (2014). The Gap Report Retrieved 18 January 2016 from www.unaids.org/en/resources/documents/2014.

Joint United Nations Programme on HIV/AIDS (UNAIDS). (2015). "15 by 15": a global target achieved. Retrieved 18 January 2016 from www.unaids.org/en/resources/documents/2015/15_by_15_a_global_target_achieved.

Kapstein, Ethan B. & Busby, Joshua W. (2013). *AIDS Drugs for All: Social Movements and Market Transformations.* Cambridge, UK: Cambridge University Press.

Keck, Margaret & Sikkink, Kathryn. (1998). *Activists Beyond Borders: Advocacy Networks in International Politics.* Ithaca, NY: Cornell University Press.

Lemanski, Charlotte. (2012). Everyday human (in)security: rescaling for the southern city. *Security Dialogue, 43*(1), 61–78.

Léonard, Sarah & Kaunert, Christian. (2011). Reconceptualizing the audience in securitization theory. In Thierry Balzacq (Ed.), *Securitization Theory: How Security Problems Emerge and Dissolve* (pp. 57–76). New York: Routledge.

Mbembe, Achille. (2001). *On the Postcolony* (A. M. Berrett, Janet Roitman, Murray Last, & Steven Rendall, Trans.). Berkeley, CA: University of California Press.

Mbembe, Achille. (2003). Necropolitics. *Public Culture, 15*(1), 11–40.

McInnes, Colin & Lee, Kelley. (2012). *Global Health and International Relations.* Cambridge, UK: Polity.

McInnes, Colin & Rushton, Simon. (2013). HIV/AIDS and securitization theory. *European Journal of International Relations, 19*(1), 115–138.

Nunes, João. (2014). *Security, Emancipation and the Politics of Health: A New Theoretical Perspective.* New York: Routledge.

Nunn, Amy, Dickman, Samuel, Natrass, Nicoli, Cornwall, Alexandra, & Gruskin, Sofia. (2012). The impacts of AIDS movements on the policy responses to HIV/AIDS in Brazil and South Africa: a comparative analysis. *Global Public Health, 7*(10), 1031–1044.

O'Manique, Colleen. (2005). The "securitisation" of HIV/AIDS in sub-Saharan Africa: a critical feminist lens. *Policy and Society, 24*(1), 24–47.

PBS. (2006, 30 May). Interview, Richard Holbrooke. *Frontline: The Age of AIDS* Retrieved June 24, 2011 from www.pbs.org/wgbh/pages/frontline/aids/interviews/holbrooke.html#ixzz1QJr3Zjvl.

Piot, Peter (2009, 23 October). (Personal interview with author).

Piot, Peter. (2012). *No Time To Lose: A Life In Pursuit of Deadly Viruses.* New York: W.W. Norton.

Risse-Kappen, Thomas. (1994). Ideas do not float freely: transnational coalitions, domestic structures, and the end of the cold war. *International Organization, 48*(2), 185–214.

Salter, Mark B. (2008). Securitization and desecuritization: a dramaturgical analysis of the Canadian Air Transport Security Authority. *Journal of International Relations and Development, 11*(4), 321–349.

Seckinelgin, Hakan. (2012). *International Security, Conflict and Gender: "HIV/AIDS is another war"*. New York: Routledge.

Shilliam, Robbie (Ed.). (2010). *International Relations and Non-Western Thought: Imperialism, Colonialism and Investigations of Global Modernity*. Abingdon: Routledge.

Smith, Malinda. (2005). The constitution of Africa as a security threat. *Review of Constitutional Studies, 10*(1), 163–206.

Smith, Raymond A. & Siplon, Patricia D. (2006). *Drugs Into Bodies: Global AIDS Treatment Activism*. Westport, CT: Praeger.

Sternberg, Steve. (2002, June 11). The Fixer takes on global AIDS; Richard Holbrooke faces the biggest challenge of his storied career. *USA Today*, D07.

Thompson, Debra. (2015). Through, against, and beyond the racial state: the transnational stratum of race. In Alexander Anievas, Nivi Manchanda & Robbie Shilliam (Eds.), *Race and Racism in International Relations: Confronting the global colour line* (pp. 44–61). New York: Routledge.

Willetts, Peter (2011). *Non-Governmental Organizations in World Politics: The Construction of Global Governance*. Abingdon: Routledge.

Williams, Michael C. (2011). The continuing evolution of securitization theory. In Thierry Balzacq (Ed.), *Securitization Theory: How Security Problems Emerge and Dissolve* (pp. 212–222). New York: Routledge.

Appendix

Research methods

Studying HIV and securitization

This is a constructivist study in which ideas, intersubjective understandings and the contested process of meaning-making over time are at the analytical core. The research approach was designed to trace linkages between speech, practices and underlying discourses to assess how, in a given bureaucratic context, these interacted to produce the idea 'HIV is a security threat', catalyse HIV securitization, and influence the evolution and outcomes of that securitization over time. Research design followed Pouliot's (2007) injunction that constructivist methodologies be inductive, interpretive and historical.

Research drew on three primary data sources: elite interviews, UN documents and other IO and government documents, and unpublished internal documents received from interviewees. Published and grey literature UN documents included newsletters published by organizations active in the early security response to HIV, programme evaluations and annual reports of UN agencies active in the security response to HIV, and transcripts of UNSC sessions. Other documents reviewed include US government documents discussing HIV as a security threat, and popular press accounts of HIV, Africa and security. Document analysis was augmented with interviews with select senior policy makers who were either current or former mid-level or senior bureaucrats in the UN system or leaders in the global response to HIV.

Following Pouliot's (2007) suggestion that "[r]esearch must begin with what it is that social agents, as opposed to analysts, believe to be real" (an approach likewise consistent with the CS framework), interview questions were designed to illuminate the origins, meaning, evolution and implications of the idea 'HIV is a security threat' in the UN system from the perspective of actors in that system, and to understand the social meaning of HIV and security for those actors. Interviews therefore included four categories of questions:

1   *What ideas were central to the construction of HIV as a security threat?*
    This entailed asking interviewees to describe how or if they regarded HIV as a security threat, and why and how they came to regard HIV in this way.

2 *Through what process was the idea 'HIV is a security threat' introduced in and diffused through the UN system and global response?* This entailed asking interviewees to recall when or from whom they first encountered this idea; what evidence sources they recalled consulting; whether there were any notable 'champions' of this idea; and to recall strategies used to inform others of the idea that HIV is a security threat.

3 *What have been the (perceived) consequences of HIV securitization?* This entailed asking interviewees about whether they had observed changes (for example, in how and where resources are allocated) since the UNSC debates on HIV, and their assessment of the impact of the debates, resolutions and associated programming.

4 *How and why did the meaning of 'HIV is a security threat' evolve over time?* This entailed asking interviewees what they had learned through positioning HIV as a security threat; whether they would, looking back, have done anything differently; what challenges they were currently experiencing; what they were currently doing to position HIV and security in particular ways; and what they anticipated, hoped or feared the security response to HIV (and the global response more generally) might look like in the future.

Interview transcripts and other documents were analysed through triangulation, process tracing, discourse analysis and content analysis. This moved analysis beyond actors' own accounts of HIV securitization, recognizing that "a study that narrowly sticks to the meanings held by actors lacks the detachment required for their historicization (where meanings come from and how they came to be) and their contextualization (how meanings relate to others and to patterns of domination). Interpretation also requires objectification" (Pouliot, 2007). Triangulation and process tracing were used to validate the sequence of events; to map the diffusion and evolution of the idea 'HIV is a security threat'; to identify contradictory accounts; and to uncover policy makers' narratives about their active role in promoting or contesting the idea 'HIV is a security threat'. As discussed in Chapters 3 and 4, discourse analysis was used to work backwards from articulated ideas to underlying assumptions and discourses by asking, 'for this articulated idea to make sense, what foundational assumptions must be at work?' Content analysis (close reading to identify ideas, themes or common categories that recurred across texts) was used to identify common themes suggesting intersubjectively shared understandings, that is, ideas operating at the level of the social or institutional environment, not just individual cognition, to give the idea 'HIV is a security threat' particular meanings and programmatic implications.

Interview process

Interviewees were identified through review of primary documents to identify participants in UNSC debates, and staff currently working in HIV and security programming, and by asking initial interviewees to suggest whom else I should speak to. Interviews were semi-structured and varied in length from 30 minutes to over two hours. Interviewees did not speak to me as official representatives of their agencies; where their organizational location is noted in the text, this is only intended to suggest how their positionality informs their perspective, and to therefore provide context useful for making sense of quoted material. Although most interviewees agreed to be interviewed with attribution, I ultimately used pseudonyms for all except two senior public figures, Peter Piot and Stephen Lewis. With the exception of Piot and Lewis, it is the organizational location and job function of interviewees, not their names, that makes their perspectives relevant; with only a few exceptions, these interviewees' names would not be known except to others working in the UN's security response to HIV, meaning that readers would not in any case be able to make sense of quoted material on the basis of name recognition.

The relatively small number of interviewees reflects that HIV and security has always been a relatively small policy and programming area in the UN, and that when interviewing elites, the number of available interviewees shrinks dramatically. There is only one Peter Piot, one Stephen Lewis. Rather than seeking wider breadth of coverage by interviewing a larger number of actors more removed from decision-making and programme implementation circles, I opted instead to interview a smaller number of influential leaders and key figures in the UN's HIV and security response.

The small number of interviewees may also be partly due to the fact that when initially contacting interviewees, I presented myself as a researcher interested in HIV and security. At that time, I was unaware of the extent to which organizational politics and boundary work had functioned to cordon off the security response to HIV and to demarcate it as a small, relatively isolated and not universally popular programming area. In responding to interview requests, some contacts who declined to be interviewed (including almost everyone whom I contacted at the WHO) explained that they were declining because they had nothing to do with HIV and security – even though in some cases they had participated in initial efforts to securitize HIV, and in almost all cases were still active in the global response to HIV. Most striking to me was that this included a representative of UN+, a network of UN staff living with HIV. This was a group of people who, it seemed to me, were significantly affected by moves to frame HIV as a security threat, in general, and by debates about provision of HIV treatment to UN staff in peacekeeping and humanitarian missions, in particular. In declining to be interviewed because they did not regard themselves or their work as part of, relevant to or affected by the security response to HIV, these contacts provided me with some of the earliest signals of the strong boundary functions played by 'security' in the UN system.

List of interviewees

To protect confidentiality, only basic information about interviewees' positions is described. The generic terms 'staff', 'manager' and 'senior manager' are used (rather than UN-system specific terms such as 'chief', 'director', 'secretary-general', etc.), where use of an interviewee's title could indicate their identity. The gender of some interviewees may also have been changed.

Peter Piot: Executive Director of UNAIDS, December 1994–December 2008
Stephen Lewis: UN Secretary-General's Special Envoy for HIV/AIDS in Africa, June 2001–December 2006; Deputy Executive Director of UNICEF, 1995–1999

UNAIDS

Keith (two interviews): Manager, Security and Humanitarian Response Unit
Rashmi: Staff, Security and Humanitarian Response Unit
Ruth: Former staff, Security and Humanitarian Response Unit
Wayne: Former senior advisor to Peter Piot

DPKO

Alex: HIV/AIDS policy staff
Eric: Former HIV/AIDS staff in a West African peacekeeping mission
Maggie: Former HIV/AIDS policy staff
Michael: Former senior leader in DPKO

UNHCR

Edward: Senior staff, Public Health and HIV Section

WHO

Charles: Manager, Department of HIV/AIDS
Geoff: Former staff, WHO Global Programme on AIDS; a former director of the Civil–Military Alliance to Combat HIV and AIDS
Gilbert (two interviews): Former staff, WHO Global Programme on AIDS; UNAIDS Uniformed Services Task Force member
Patrick: Former advisor to senior WHO officials

UNFPA

Cindy: Staff, Humanitarian Response Unit
June: Former manager, Humanitarian Response Unit

Reference

Pouliot, V. 2007. "Sobjectivism": Toward a Constructivist Methodology. *International Studies Quarterly*, 51, 359–384.

Index

Page numbers in *italics* denote tables, those in **bold** denote figures.

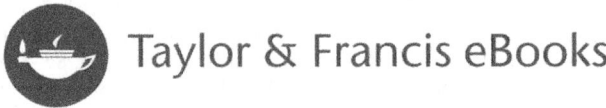
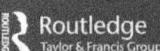